# Risk Stratification: A Practical Guide for Clinicians

Risk stratification is a statistical process by which quality of care can be assessed independently of patient case-mix. Evaluation of risk-adjusted patient outcome has become an important part of managed-care contracting in some markets, and risk-adjusted outcome rates for hospitals are being reported more frequently in the popular press and on the Internet. This book, written by a statistician and two surgeons for a clinical audience, is a practical guide to the process of risk stratification and does not require or assume an extensive mathematical background. It describes the rationale and assumptions for risk stratification, and provides information on evaluating the quality of various published risk-stratification studies. Numerous practical examples using real clinical data help to illustrate risk stratification in health-care. The book also serves as a step-by-step guide to the production and dissemination of risk-adjusted outcome results for local programs.

**Charles C. Miller III** is Associate Professor and Chief of the Division of Clinical Research in the Department of Cardiothoracic and Vascular Surgery at the University of Texas Health Sciences Center at Houston.
**Michael J. Reardon** is Professor of Surgery and Director of the Residency Program in the Division of Cardiothoracic Surgery at Baylor College of Medicine, Houston.
**Hazim J. Safi** is Professor and Chairman of the Department of Cardiothoracic and Vascular Surgery at the University of Texas Health Sciences Center at Houston.

# Risk Stratification

## A Practical Guide for Clinicians

Charles C. Miller III
The University of Texas, Houston

Michael J. Reardon
Baylor College of Medicine, Houston

Hazim J. Safi
The University of Texas, Houston

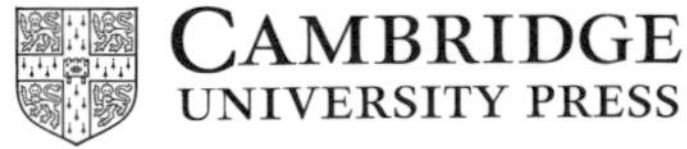
CAMBRIDGE
UNIVERSITY PRESS

PUBLISHED BY THE PRESS SYNDICATE OF THE UNIVERSITY OF CAMBRIDGE
The Pitt Building, Trumpington Street, Cambridge, United Kingdom

CAMBRIDGE UNIVERSITY PRESS
The Edinburgh Building, Cambridge CB2 2RU, UK
40 West 20th Street, New York, NY 10011-4211, USA
10 Stamford Road, Oakleigh, VIC 3166, Australia
Ruiz de Alarcón 13, 28014 Madrid, Spain
Dock House, The Waterfront, Cape Town 8001, South Africa

http://www.cambridge.org



First published 2001

Printed in the United Kingdom at the University Press, Cambridge

*Typeface* Minion 11/14.5 pt. *System* QuarkXPress™ [SE]

*A catalogue record for this book is available from the British Library*

ISBN 0 521 66945 6 paperback

**C.C.M.**

**For Kate**
**and in memory of Joe Rodarte, mentor and friend**

**M.J.R.**

**For Robin, Robin Heather, and Rebecca**

**H.J.S.**

**For my Mother, Aminah**

Houston, Texas, 2000

# Contents

# Preface

This book is a practical guide to the quantitative estimation and stratification of medical risk. It is not about legal risk, or about the business risk that is associated with capitated insurance plans. Although some of the concepts described in the pages to follow could provide useful information for evaluating aspects of the risk pertinent to other professional domains, we will not discuss such applications in this book. Medical risk, as we define it here, is the probability that a specific kind of event or outcome will occur following or in connection with a medical intervention. The intervention and the outcome can be anything, as long as they can be measured with reasonable accuracy, so that a relationship between them can be evaluated.

Risk stratification is a branch of clinical research, but it differs from classic efficacy-oriented medical research in an important way. Rather than evaluating the efficacy of a treatment, it determines whether events that occur in a local population are accounted for by the risk factors in that population. Said another way, risk stratification determines whether events, such as deaths following surgery, infections in the hospital, etc., that occur in a particular population can be explained by risk factors that are known to produce such events. If more events occur in a population than would be expected based on risk factors, some other source of the excess event rate is inferred to be present in the population. In a formal risk-stratification study, a local population is standardized by comparison to the well-known risk factors of an established model. An example from the literature on coronary bypass would be to take the risk factors established by the New York State Department of Health's published logistic regression model and apply the weights of those risk factors to the prevalences of the same risk factors in a local clinic population. This process would produce a prediction of the number of events (in this example in-hospital deaths following coronary bypass) that would be likely to occur in the local clinic population on the basis of that population's risk factor profile.

We will deal with risk adjustment and risk stratification mainly as these are described by multivariate mathematical models, because such models are ubiquitous in the literature and have become the standard in risk prediction technology. We will not, generally speaking, dwell on the underlying mathematical aspects of risk modeling, because an understanding of the mathematics is not really necessary for the application of these models to data and interpretation of the results. Instead, we will focus on the assumptions required to justify the use of such models, and on the data required to make them work. We will use examples to describe situations in which certain types of data can be used to predict certain types of outcomes, and will provide SAS code that does the calculations. We will also show sample output from computer runs of the examples, and will show how to interpret the findings. In most circumstances, readers should be able to substitute their own data into the examples and come up with correct results.

Readers of this book will not need to have advanced mathematical training. A grasp of basic algebra and a willingness to put a bit of thought into the problems are all that is required. This book is intended for three major types of consumers. First, clinicians who want to understand the process of risk stratification and to understand what the numbers compiled from their own data might mean. Chapters 1 and 5 provide information on the assumptions and limitations of risk models and describe important issues such as data quality. For these readers, the book will be a primer in the methods and an explanation of how the process works. Second, people charged with development of a risk-stratification program (office managers, case managers, physicians, unlucky medical students, etc.), who need a step-by-step cookbook for putting together a program, will also find the book useful. These readers should read the book all the way through and use it as a shop manual that shows how to build a program from the ground up. Third, people at any level (MPH physicians, office managers who were math undergraduates, etc.) who understand the big picture issues but lack a small piece of the puzzle will also find what they need here. For these readers, the book will serve as a central reference that will provide the missing pieces that are unavailable elsewhere in the medical literature. Chapters 4 and 6 explain the computational details and the conversion of risk factor data to numbers of expected cases using logistic regression and direct standardization methods.

It has been our intent to write a book that is both detailed and flexible enough to provide multiple levels of information for several types of reader. In the pages that follow, we will describe the concept of probability, and the estimation of probability using published models or other models based on data. We will show how the presence of various patient characteristics leads to predictions about individual outcome, and how the distribution of characteristics in populations leads to estimates of population risk. We will describe the process of risk adjustment, by which actual outcome rates are interpreted with regard to expectations based on risk models. Finally, we will discuss the limitations of risk prediction and risk adjustment, and provide a discussion of application and interpretation of risk model output.

We are grateful to our teachers and students, who over the years have taught us many nuances of clinical research, and have demanded that we justify and explain our thinking carefully in return. Among these are our former trainees Dr Dan Root and Rebecca Prince, who read maddeningly rough and disjointed early drafts of several chapters, and made many useful comments on the manuscript. We are particularly grateful to Dr Gerald Adams, an *ad hoc* consultant who provided a detailed and thoughtful review of the entire first draft of the manuscript, and who made many useful comments. The work of all these readers has greatly improved the quality of the manuscript. Any errors that remain after the careful readings of our colleagues remain solely our responsibility. We are also grateful to Jennifer Goodrick and John O'Donnell, our research nurses, who put many hours into designing programs and collecting data, and for making the daily nuts and bolts of an extensive risk-stratification program work. We also express special thanks to Amy Wirtz Newland, our Departmental editor, who, with no formal training in statistics and little in clinical research, suffered through every single word of the manuscript. She demanded that we illuminate the many corners we had left dark in the glossing-over which comes with too many years of using these concepts on a daily basis, and made many needed changes to our awkward scientific prose. Finally, we are grateful to our colleagues and especially to our families for their patience with us during the writing, and we are also grateful to our editors at Cambridge University Press, Jo-Ann Strangis and Peter Silver, for their support and enthusiasm.

# Introduction

The mathematical prediction and stratification of medical risk has received increased attention in recent years, as interest in comparing and rating health care provider organizations has grown. Some of this interest has been driven by competition between organizations that wish to show their own results as compared to those of their competitors down the street or across the country. Some of the interest has come through governmental oversight and the declaration of performance standards based on risk expectations. The state of New York, for example, influences the practice patterns of physicians who perform coronary bypass operations by publishing comprehensive statewide risk stratification program results (1). Perhaps the greatest interest among individual practices and institutions has been developed in response to questions posed by managed care companies, as risk-adjusted results have become a more important part of contracting. There are many reasons for collecting data on local performance and considering the implementation of some sort of risk stratification program in nearly every clinical practice organization.

A feature common to all risk stratification, regardless of its ultimate purpose, is that it compares outcomes from a particular institution or clinical practice with those of a recognized standard. In making such comparisons, risk stratification considers risk factor distributions that may not be identical between the populations being compared, and uses the risk factors to explain some of the variation in the outcomes of one population based on expectations derived from another. The process requires that a risk model of some sort, which serves as the standard for comparison, be applied to local risk factor data. From this, the number (or the percent in some cases) of outcome events that would have been expected in the local population based on the risk factors in that population is computed. The resulting number is the number of cases expected in the local population, adjusted for their risk factors, if the care provided to them were identical to that provided to the standard population. Consider the following simplified example. Imagine a standard group that has 20 patients, one of whom dies following a particular kind of operation. Suppose that this patient dies because of a cardiac problem; say, a very low left ventricular ejection fraction. If we had another group of 20 comparable patients, and one had a low ejection fraction, we might expect one death in the second group as well, based on our experience with the first group, all other things being equal. If we actually observed five deaths in the second population instead of the one death we had expected, we might be faced with the possibility that a problem exists with the care provided to the second group of patients. Risk stratification helps us get an idea of whether a particular outcome is in line with what we would expect it to be based on underlying patient risk. Although no predictions are perfect, and these examples are oversimplified for purposes of illustration, predictions based on risk models can be very helpful for informing our expectations. The point is that we do have tools for making good predictions, and if we use them properly and we get good measurements, we can reduce the uncertainty of prediction a good deal. Risk stratification is nothing more than a way of formalizing the often heard claim that "our results are not as good as those of institution X down the street because we treat sicker patients". By risk stratifying we adjust out the population effects of risk factors by controlling for them mathematically. This allows for "level playing field" comparisons between populations, which are much easier to understand and interpret than "crude" or unadjusted comparisons. In the pages that follow we will describe the rationale and many of the technical details of risk stratification, and will show how a comprehensive program of risk analysis can be assembled by clinicians at their own institutions.

## Comparing care across institutions

Use of risk-adjusted comparisons for evaluating quality of care across institutions, and even among physicians, is a large and growing practice.

The scope and level of detail of such evaluations vary greatly, as does the use to which the evaluations are put. The New York State Department of Health collects patient-level, clinical data on each patient who undergoes coronary bypass grafting in the state. The Department then publishes reports that profile the risk-adjusted mortality of hospitals and of individual surgeons. The Society of Thoracic Surgeons maintains a nationwide voluntary-participation registry and risk-adjustment database on cardiac surgery that uses extensive clinical data (2). Health-care provider-evaluation corporations have also begun to make extremely large comparisons of risk-adjusted mortality and length of stay using administrative data. The Medicare Provider Analysis and Review (MEDPAR) system contains data on principal diagnosis, secondary comorbid diagnoses, and some limited demographic information about every Medicare patient who is hospitalized for a Medicare diagnosis in the United States. Risk analyses based on this type of data have appeared on Internet sites, in popular press articles and many other forms of publication in recent years, and many of these publications have ranked hospitals on the basis of their risk-adjusted performance. Administrative data are far less detailed and less accurate than clinical data for this activity, but studies based on administrative data are the largest and most prevalent studies today because of easy public access to Medicare data files.

Comparisons between institutions are only as good as the data on which they are based, and the interpretation of such comparisons is a major factor in their usefulness. We spend some time on the differences between administrative and clinical data-based research in Chapter 5, and cover issues regarding their interpretation and use.

## Risk benchmarking for following care over time

Risk stratification can be used within institutions or within individual practice organizations to measure the process of care and to follow changes in outcome over time. We have found this to be extremely useful in our own environs, and have evaluated many of the changes we have made over the years in the process of care using risk-stratified comparisons. Changes in surgical technique, supportive care and other aspects of the care process can be evaluated informally using data that are corrected for fluctuations in the underlying risk profile of the population over time, so that actual changes rather than apparent ones due to risk factor changes can be studied. Use of risk-stratified data for this purpose is best confined to the intellectual domain of "hypothesis-generating" studies however, because traditional clinical research studies are always warranted where formal evaluation of new treatments is at issue.

## Predicting risk for individual patients

Calculation of expected risk for an individual patient prior to a medical intervention can be done using risk-stratification equations. This can be very useful for making treatment decisions, preparing for postintervention care, and for helping the patient and family to make informed choices about treatment options. Quantitative expectations about individual patient risk can be very helpful in the consent process, and can also be very useful for fine-tuning the care plans for patients. An awareness not only that a patient is *at* increased risk of diabetes-related morbidity following surgery, for example, but also an awareness of *how much* risk that patient faces can assist in care planning and quality by activating different intensities of specific kinds of care based on risk. Some institutions have begun to experiment with using risk-stratification data to create dynamic clinical care pathways for individual patients. Rather than having a single care pathway for all heart failure patients, for example, a hospital might put one heart failure patient on one pathway if he or she had significant pulmonary edema, and another patient on a different pathway if he or she had a low ejection fraction but no frank symptoms. This is an area that is ripe with opportunities for research, and for the development of dramatic improvements in the efficiency of health-care delivery.

## A note on terms

We use the term "multivariate" rather loosely here to mean any statistical analysis that uses more than one independent variable (risk factor variable) to explain an event (outcome). This usage is common and is widely familiar to readers. The term "multivariate" has historically been used by mathematical statisticians as a technical term in regression analysis to denote the simultaneous solution of a model for both more than one *dependent* (outcome) variable and more than one *independent* (predictor) variable. This comes mainly from the analysis of variance literature, where the technical acronym MANOVA is used to represent multivariate analysis of variance, which is a multiple *independent and dependent* variable statistical method. In deference to this historical usage, many authors continue to use the terms "multiple" and "multivariable" when referring to regression analyses with more than one independent variable but only one dependent variable, specifically to avoid using the term "multivariate" in this context. In practice today, because multiple dependent-variable models are very uncommonly encountered in the applied literature, the term "doubly multivariate" is usually applied to models with multiple dependent and independent variables. For the sake of grammatical variety we use the terms "multiple", "multivariable" and "multivariate" interchangeably to denote the use of a multiple *independent* variable model with a single dependent variable. We do not cover multiple dependent variable logistic models in this book, which are an advanced topic for another day. Similarly, we use "risk" and "probability" interchangeably, to mean long-term relative frequency. Readers will find definitions for most important terms in the margins of the text as the terms are introduced. Where terms have specific technical usage, we state the definition explicitly in the text.

The field of risk stratification is vast and the quality and focus of studies in the field are broad and variable. It is our intent here to provide a lucid narrative and examples that will help the reader to understand, apply and interpret the concepts. Risk stratification has many useful applications as well as many limitations. Well-researched and constructed risk models can help us sort out the effects of underlying patient characteristics on outcome and can provide much better information on the effects of care than would otherwise be available. As long as the limitations to what these models can do and should be used for are respected, risk-stratification models can tell us a great deal about our patients and our own processes of care.

## REFERENCES

1 Hannan EL, Siu AL, Kumar D, Kilburn H, Jr., Chassin MR. The decline in coronary artery bypass graft surgery mortality in New York State. The role of surgeon volume. *JAMA* 1995; **273**: 209–13.

2 Grover FL. The Society of Thoracic Surgeons national database: current status and future directions. *Ann Thorac Surg* 1999; **68**: 367–73.

# 1

# Risk

Risk stratification, although somewhat complex mathematically in its more advanced forms, is relatively easy to understand in its principles. In this chapter, we provide introductory information, which describes the rationale that underlies many of the statistical methods that are used in risk assessment and stratification. In order to avoid the mathematical intimidation that so often accompanies these problems, we have attempted to avoid long theoretical discussions and the pages of equations that go along with them in favor of heuristic illustrations. Some things, like the difference between odds and probability, are fundamental concepts that can only be simplified so much. Nonetheless, we have tried to make the examples as clear as they can be. Readers who are already familiar with the concepts of probability and odds, and who understand univariate and multivariate techniques can skip this chapter. Those who are less familiar with the concepts or who have never interpreted a logistic regression model will benefit from reading it and we recommend that they do so. It will pay off when we go through the practice of interpreting the models in later chapters.

## Populations and samples

**Population**
A group, too large to measure, whose characteristics are understood by inference.

Before embarking on a discussion of what risk is and how it is interpreted, we should go over the concepts of population and sample briefly, because these concepts form the basis of statistical inference as we will be using it in this book. A *population* is a group that we want to know something about – say, the population of all men aged 75 who require coronary bypass surgery. We might want to know what the risk of in-hospital mortality following coronary surgery is for this population, so we could find out what the risk factors are and see whether we can do anything to mitigate the risk and improve survival. Because we cannot possibly measure risk on every single 75-year-old man who has coronary surgery, it is necessary for us to make our measurements on a *sample* of the population. Ideally, because 75-year-old men in general have physiological similarities, the experience of a sample will reflect the overall experience of the population. That is, we will use data collected from a sample to make an *inference* about a population, most of whom we will never actually see. All clinical medicine is based on the idea that it is possible to learn something from one group of patients and apply it to another. That is, inference-making from samples is not just for statisticians – population inferences are the foundation of clinical practice. If each patient responded differently to the same medical treatment, outcomes would be wildly unpredictable, and Medicine as we know it today would not exist. Fortunately, patients tend to respond similarly and therefore predictably to treatment. Risk stratification relies fundamentally on this long-standing clinical wisdom, and adds various quantitative features to help us get a better handle on the magnitude, variability, and predictors of risk.

**Sample**
A subset of a population on which measurements are made. Inferences about populations are drawn from measurements made on samples.

Summary measures computed from sample data are called *statistics.* Proportions, percents, averages, medians, standard deviations, and other methods of summarizing samples are statistics. Statistics are used to estimate population *parameters*, which are the corresponding values of the variables measured in the sample that we would expect to exist in the population that we ultimately want to know something about. For example, when we measure the in-hospital mortality rate that occurs after coronary bypass surgery, we do it partly to summarize past experience, and this summarization is made using information from a sample. But we also measure in-hospital mortality because it is our best guide to what will happen in the future. Predictions are not about members of a sample, but are about members of the population that we know we will see but have yet to measure. We can use the same statistic, such as the proportion of coronary bypass deaths in our hospital's recent experience, to provide both a sample summary and a population prediction. We will come back to this business of extrapolating to populations from samples in detail later, but it is worth making the following cautionary

**Statistics**
The summary result of a measurement or measurements made on a sample. Statistics provide estimates of population parameters.

**Parameters**
Unknown characteristics of a population that we estimate with statistics.

statement at the outset. Since all numerical operations are carried out on samples, the characteristics of the samples that are selected will affect the inferences we make about larger populations. Biased samples will lead us to incorrect conclusions about the population that we ultimately wish to understand. We will cover bias in detail later on, but, briefly, a bias is any systematic abnormality in a sample that causes it to deviate from the characteristics of the population from which it is drawn. For example, a study of risk factors for lung cancer might be biased if patients are afraid to tell a judgmental interviewer about their heavy smoking in the past. If people downplay their smoking but smoking is really a major risk factor, differences in smoking behavior between people who get lung cancer and those who do not will appear to be smaller than they actually are, and smoking will consequently appear falsely to be unimportant as a risk factor. Since samples are supposed to represent populations, biased samples do not do a good job of representation. Bias in the samples from which we draw estimates will be reflected in any expectations we develop about the larger population in the future.

## Probability and risk

**Probability**
The chance that an event will occur, expressed as the frequency with which an event has arisen on previous occasions under similar circumstances relative to the occurrence of other potential outcomes.

Numerous ways exist to describe *probability* but, unless otherwise noted, in this book we will use the statistical concept of probability as frequency. By frequency we mean simply the number of events. More specifically, we characterize probability as long-term relative frequency, or the frequency with which a certain event would be expected to occur over many repeated observations over time. Our best estimate of the probability that an event will occur in a given situation is the frequency with which such an event has arisen in the past under similar circumstances, *relative to the occurrence of other potential outcomes.* If, for example, on average, three of every 100 patients undergoing coronary bypass died in the hospital sometime following surgery, we would say that the probability of in-hospital mortality following coronary bypass is three percent. Percent is a commonly used relative frequency, from the Latin *per centum* – per hundred, and in this case is the number of events per hundred cases. So we evaluate the frequency of events (deaths) in relationship to the whole group (100 patients), which includes the survivors as well. Raw frequency that is not standardized to a population denominator would tell us very little. We would view three deaths quite differently if they occurred in a group of 100 patients than we would if they occurred in a group of four. So we can use relative frequency estimates gained from past experience to estimate the probability of future events. The ability to do this is the basis of *risk* stratification, and it is the discipline's fundamental assumption. If we knew nothing about a patient who was coming to the hospital other than that he or she was scheduled for coronary bypass surgery tomorrow, we would estimate, based on our past experience, that the risk of hospital mortality following the procedure would be three percent. Long-term relative frequency of past events provides the best information on what future experience will be like.

**Risk**
Probability – or long-term relative frequency.

In practice, when our patient is admitted to the hospital we will know more about him or her than simply that a coronary bypass operation is scheduled for tomorrow morning. Most likely, we will know the patient's age and gender, the extent of the coronary disease, important cardiac function information such as left ventricular ejection fraction, and their medical history for such co-existing problems as diabetes mellitus and renal dysfunction. Patient characteristics of this type are known as *risk factors.* They are characteristics which, in past experience, have been observed to modify the risk of coronary bypass operations. Since we like to learn from experience, and since human physiological responses are somewhat predictable, these risk factors should be useful to modify our expectations for the future as well.

**Risk factors**
Patient characteristics that modify the probability that a specific event will occur in that patient.

While we might say that the hospital mortality risk for the average coronary bypass patient is three percent, we can sharpen our expectations to some degree by taking a patient's individual risk factors into account. Predictions based on risk factors require that we accept the assumption that hospital mortality does not occur entirely at random in these patients. That is, certain characteristics predispose people to hospital death, and the deaths can be explained, above and beyond some basic level of uncertainty, by the presence of the risk factors. A basic level of uncertainty means simply that we cannot make completely accurate predictions every time no matter how good our information. Biological organisms, like humans, vary somewhat in their outcome experience in ways that we cannot explain. Some patients with very high risk profiles survive, in defiance of our expectations. Likewise, it is occasionally the case that patients who appear to be at low risk die unexpectedly. Predictions are only estimates of risk based on past experience in similar circumstances. Nothing can give us perfect prediction of future events. It is also worth pointing out that not all risk factors increase risk – some of them mitigate it. For example, pregnant women who take vitamin supplements containing folic acid reduce the risk of neural tube defects in their offspring (1). In this case, vitamin use is a risk factor, but it is a protective one. It is a risk factor that has a downward modifying effect on risk.

Intuitively, back to the coronary bypass example, we can easily understand that a 75-year-old male patient with four-vessel disease, a myocardial infarction in the past seven days, diabetes mellitus, renal failure and a left ventricular ejection fraction of 25 percent would have a different hospital mortality expectation than a 50-year-old male with single-vessel disease and no other risk factors. The question is, how much difference do the risk factors make, and how do we sort out their relative contributions to the overall risk? We start by looking at the case of a single risk factor. Figure 1.1 shows the risk of hospital mortality for males distributed by age. The computations for the risk estimates shown in the figure are somewhat complex. We will cover them in greater detail later in the book, but the figure itself is easy to understand. As age goes up, so does hospital mortality following coronary bypass surgery, particularly beyond the age of 70. Although the concept of increasing risk with increasing age would seem obvious to the most casual observer, the information contained in the risk figure gives us something casual observation does not. It gives us quantitative information about the magnitude of hospital mortality risk and how that risk is modified by the patient's age.

## Risk and odds

So far we have talked about risk as being equal to probability, which we have defined as long-term relative frequency. The calculation of relative frequency for a single outcome in a defined population is straightforward. In our previous example of three coronary bypass hospital deaths in 100 patients we divide the number of deaths (3) by the population size (100), and multiply that proportion by 100 to get the number expected per hundred (percent). But, before we go too much further, a discussion of odds, probability, and their relationship is warranted. This will be extremely helpful in interpreting the results of some of the multivariate formulas we discuss later on.

Major surgery (or, more accurately, the disease that creates the need for the surgery) subjects every patient who undergoes it to a certain amount of risk. Therefore, in our example group of 100 patients, we can think of each of the 100 operations as representing an independent chance, with the outcome of the chance being survival or death. The probability calculation we just did shows that there are three chances in 100 that a patient who undergoes a coronary bypass operation will die in the hospital. Based on the experience of our sample, and, in keeping with our concept of probability as *long-term* relative frequency, we would make the generalization that, on average, of every 100 chances taken in the overall population, three will result in a death. For now we are setting aside any notions of risk associated with the patients' clinical conditions, and are thinking of the risk as a random phenomenon – as though the patients were drawing straws.

**Odds**
The chance that an event will occur versus the chance that it will not.

*Odds* are related to probability, but are not the same thing. The terms are often used interchangeably in casual conversation, but there are technical differences that are quite important for risk stratification as we will see later on. Odds express the likelihood that someone will die (three in our example) against the likelihood that they will not (100 at risk minus 3 dead = 97 survivors). So while the *probability* that someone will die is 3/100, or three percent, the *odds* of dying in the hospital following a coronary bypass are 3:97. Reducing the fraction and rounding the decimals, we would say that the odds are roughly 1:32 *against* survival, or 32:1 *in favor* of survival. We say that odds are against an outcome when the odds of the outcome's occurrence are *less* than 1:1. In our example, the odds of *non-survival* are only one in 32, so the odds are less than 1:1. Alternatively, we would say that the odds favor an outcome when the chances of the outcome are *greater* than 1:1. Here, odds of survival are 32:1 – much greater than 1:1. Ultimately, probability is what we are after, because that is what we will use to make comparisons between populations, but we have to get there via odds for mathematical reasons in some circumstances, which we will explain in detail later on. Odds can be converted to probability by the formula:

Equation 1.1

$$p = o/(1 + o)$$

where $p$ = probability and $o$ = odds.

So in our example, odds are 3/97 = 0.030928, and probability computed from equation 1.1 is 0.030928/1.030928 = 0.03, or three percent – the same as we got from the original 3/100 computation. The difference between 0.0309 and 0.03 looks so trivial that many readers may wonder why we even cover it. In truth, probability and odds are quite close for *rare events*. But in circumstances where the populations are small relative to the events (i.e., the events are common), the differences between odds expressed as a fraction and probability can be quite large. For example, in a case where 50 deaths occurred in 100 patients, the probability would be 50/100 = 1/2 = 0.50. Odds, on the other hand, would be 50:50, or 1:1 or 1/1 = 1.0. Another important difference to keep in mind is that probability is constrained by zero and one. A probability of zero means something never happens, and a probability of one means it happens every time. Odds, on the other hand, are not constrained by zero and one. As any lottery player should know, odds can be tens of millions (or more) to one.

**Event**
A patient outcome.

Traditionally, in epidemiological studies, risk and odds are calculated to estimate different kinds of effects. Risk is computed for incidence data to estimate the probability that a subject will get a disease given an *exposure.* An exposure in epidemiological terms is a risk factor as we have been using the term – anything that modifies the risk of an outcome. "Disease", as used by epidemiologists, is the same as we have used outcome. It can be a death after coronary surgery, a neural tube defect in a live-born child, or any other event we would like to study. *Incidence* is the rate at which new cases of an outcome arise in a population. For example, the 30-day cumulative incidence of mortality following coronary bypass surgery might be three percent, and it might accumulate to three percent at the rate of one percent per ten days. Incidence always refers to new cases arising in a population over time, and only among people who are at risk for developing the outcome. People who have a particular disease or outcome at the time they are identified by a study

**Exposure**
A term used in epidemiology that refers to a risk factor. It can be a medical treatment or an environmental exposure, among other things.

are not considered to be at risk for the disease, and do not become part of the non-diseased cohort that begins an incidence study. If we wanted to study risk factors for conversion of human immunodeficiency virus (HIV) seropositivity in a population of adults, for example, we would exclude people who were found to have antibodies to HIV at baseline screening. Such people would not be at risk for developing the disease since they already have it, and their participation in a study would not contribute useful information about the *onset* rate of seropositivity.

Odds, on the other hand, are calculated for *prevalence* data to estimate the likelihood that a person who has a disease was exposed to something thought to have caused it. Here, again, exposure is risk factor and disease is outcome. Prevalence, though, describes all prevalent cases of a disease at the time of study, without regard (with some exceptions) to when the disease came on. So another way we might think of an HIV seropositivity study would be to find a group of people who are seropositive and a group who are not, and compare risk factors between the groups to see what is different. Incidence studies look forward in time to the rate of onset of the outcome. Prevalence studies look backward in time from a prevalent disease to something thought to have caused it. Ratios between groups, exposed versus unexposed for risk and diseased versus non-diseased for odds, are taken to estimate the magnitude of an association between risk factors and disease. Risk ratio (or relative risk) and odds ratio are the terms used to describe these measures of association. We present a brief sketch of the epidemiological use of risk and odds only to illuminate their differences. Much more discussion at this point will distract us from what we want to say about risk and odds for our immediate purposes in this chapter. We will save further elaboration on these points for a later chapter. For now, suffice it to say that risk studies are nearly always concerned with incidence data, because their goal is to predict the onset of new outcomes in future experience. However, probability of outcome is often expressed in terms of odds and odds ratios in risk studies, because incidence is very efficiently modeled as the prevalence of new cases over a period of time. There are numerous technical considerations that govern the application of these methods for expressing likelihood in such studies. We will discuss study designs for incidence and prevalence studies in detail in later chapters.

## Risk and a single risk factor

Calculation of risk for a one-variable (survive or not, as in the previous examples) population is simple, as we have seen. In the one-variable scenario, the outcome can be assumed to be randomly distributed within the population – as though the population members were drawing straws. As modifiers of an outcome probability, risk factors account for a proportion of the total variance in the outcome, and by doing so reduce the amount of random variation contributing to the total variation in outcome. While some random variation will always be present, risk factors properly described can account for a good deal of it. Even in the presence of risk factors, we can think of the population as drawing straws, but those with more extensive risk factors will be *more likely* to draw a short straw than will those at lower risk.

Not all risk factors are equal in their influence on the probability of an outcome. Consequently, some determination of which risk factors to consider needs to be made before estimates of multivariate risk are attempted. The process of evaluating risk factors involves measurements of the association between risk factors and outcome. When we are looking for association between a single risk factor and an outcome, we usually want to use what is known as a contingency table approach, where we would divide our sample into four groups: (1) those with both the outcome and the risk factor; (2) those with the outcome but not the risk factor; (3) those with the risk factor but not the outcome; and (4) those with neither the risk factor nor the outcome. The reason for doing this is to determine whether the outcome is more likely to occur when the risk factor is present than when it is absent. Consider the following example. We know that patients who come to the operating room for coronary bypass surgery in congestive heart failure (CHF) with active dilated cardiomyopathy are very sick patients. Suppose we hypothesize that patients who have symptomatic CHF at the time of surgery have a higher expected mortality than patients who do not come to surgery with this problem. In order to examine this hypothesis, we would arrange data into the four categories we previously mentioned, which are shown in Table 1.1.

In Table 1.1 we have a hypothetical (not real patient data – for

**Table 1.1** Contingency table for hospital death by preoperative congestive heart failure (CHF)

| | CHF | No CHF | |
|---|---|---|---|
| Died in hospital | 10 (10%) | 3 (3%) | 13 |
| Did not die in hospital | 90 | 97 | 187 |
| | 100 | 100 | 200 |

Probability in CHF group = 10/100 = 0.10 = 10%
Probability in no-CHF group = 3/100 = 0.03 = 3%
Odds in CHF group = 10/90 = 0.1111 = 9: 1 in favor of survival
Odds in no-CHF group = 3/97 = 0.0309 = 32: 1 in favor of survival
Odds ratio = 0.1111/0.0309 = 3.59

illustration only) group of 200 patients, 100 of whom had active CHF at the time of surgery and 100 of whom did not. Of the 100 with CHF, ten died in hospital, compared to three deaths in the 100 without CHF. We mentioned above that the data are divided into four groups, represented by the four cells of the table. The upper left cell contains data for ten patients who had both the risk factor (CHF) and the outcome (hospital death). The cell to the right represents three patients who did not have the risk factor but had the outcome anyway. The lower left cell contains data for 90 people who had the risk factor but not the outcome, and the last cell shows data for 97 people who had neither the risk factor nor the outcome. In parentheses below the numbers in the top two cells are the percents of people at risk in each risk factor group (with and without) who had the outcome. We see that ten percent of patients in the CHF group died in hospital, and three percent of the patients without CHF also died in hospital. Computation of probabilities, percents, and odds are shown below the table. Showing odds in gambler's notation (referenced to one) involves reducing the fraction by dividing both sides by the smaller number. So odds on 10 of 90 in the CHF group becomes 10/10:90/10 = 1:9. Because death is the rare event, we arrange the odds to be in favor of survival rather than death, so we say that the odds are 9:1 in favor of survival for the CHF group. Simply eyeballing the data thus arrayed suggests that hospital mortality after coronary bypass surgery is higher in the CHF group than in the non-CHF group. Statistical tests exist to determine whether this difference is significant, but we will cover those in Chapter 6. We show examples in this chapter only to give a flavor of how the process works.

Unfortunately, once a determination has been made that a risk factor is associated with an outcome (i.e., the outcome is more common when a risk factor is present than when it is absent), there is almost always some remaining question about whether it is the risk factor itself or something else related to the risk factor that is the source of the association. In our CHF example, it may be true that people who present with CHF at the time of operation have more severe heart disease. This might be due to hypertrophic cardiomyopathy, to a recent myocardial infarction and consequent wall motion abnormalities, etc. Other explanations for outcome probabilities that are correlated with both the risk factor (CHF) and the outcome (coronary bypass mortality) being studied can *confound* the relationship between the main risk factor and the outcome. *Confounding* occurs when an extraneous variable explains a portion of the outcome probability that is not captured by the risk factor being evaluated. Multivariate studies, which can use mathematical techniques to partition the relative contributions of risk factor variables to outcome probabilities, are usually needed to sort out the relationships between multiple possible risk factors and outcomes.

**Confounding**
Mixing of the effects of two variables with regard to a third variable.

## Risk and multiple risk factors

Though the idea that risk factors will modify outcome probability is easily understood, and the calculation of the influence of a single risk factor is straightforward, it is not as simple to calculate probabilities when considering multiple risk factors. In practice, and particularly in biological systems, most factors that contribute to risk are not independent of one another.

Lack of independence between risk factors with respect to outcome can lead to confounding. Confounding can occur in more than one dimension (between more than two risk factors) at a time. For example, we know that patients who come to the operating room with CHF have failing hearts. This heart failure can be due to dilated cardiomyopathy caused by long-standing hypertension. Or it can be caused by a myocardial infarction, which may be caused by coronary atherosclerosis, which may be caused by hypertension, diabetes mellitus, and advanced age. Each of these factors is a risk factor in its own right, but taken together they all conspire to increase the mortality after an operation for coronary heart disease. In this sense, they are certainly not independent (i.e., they are inter-related). A group of univariate tests on each of them would not tell us anything about how these factors work together to modify overall risk. We would say, then, that the results of univariate risk factor studies that examine each of the variables individually are subject to confounding by the other related factors.

In epidemiological studies and even clinical trials, where the goal ordinarily is to look at one risk factor or treatment and adjust away the effects of others, confounding is more of a concern than it is in the kind of multiple risk factor studies that are the subject of this book. When we are looking for cause–effect relationships attributable to a single predictor variable in a clinical trial or epidemiological study, we wish to separate that predictor from other influential variables so we can interpret its *independent* effect. That is, if we were just interested in the effect of CHF on coronary bypass mortality, we would still need to measure and control for other things that are related to both CHF and mortality following this procedure; for example, high blood pressure, myocardial infarction, and so on. We would need to do this to avoid confusing the effect of CHF with the effects of the other predictors that may have caused it or may be correlated with both CHF and mortality after bypass surgery in a non-causal way. When we wish, in contrast to epidemiological or clinical trial studies, to identify *all* the important risk factors (as we do in risk-stratification studies) that work together to modify the risk of an outcome, the term "confounding" is less appropriate. In the risk-stratification situation, we do not care about CHF any more than we do about myocardial infarction – we are not trying to isolate the effect of one variable over another. Rather, we need to account mathematically for the joint predictive efficacy of all the variables together in order to get the most sensitive and specific predictor of the outcome.

To interpret the contributions of co-existing risk factors correctly as they apply to outcome, it is necessary to make an adjustment for the lack of independence between the risk factor variables. The aggregate probability of the risk factors depends on the way the factors relate to one another, and also the way they relate jointly to the outcome. The outcome probability in this case is said to be *conditional* on the risk factors. Numerous methods exist for dealing with the need to account for conditional probabilities, including stratified analysis, multivariable regression techniques such as logistic regression and classification and regression tree (CART) models, neural networks, and Bayesian approaches. Logistic regression has numerous desirable properties and is very widely used in the risk-stratification literature. Throughout this book, we will focus on logistic regression analysis, which is a powerful technique that can be used to accumulate risk that arises from multiple, and not necessarily independent, predictive factors.

Logistic regression analysis is a mathematical modeling technique that describes a relationship between one or more risk factors and the conditional probability of an outcome. Like linear regression analysis, which we anticipate will be familiar to most readers, logistic regression models a response variable (also known as a dependent variable) on one or more predictor variables (also known as independent variables). For logistic analysis, the response variable will ultimately be outcome probability, and the predictor variables will be risk factors. We say that the response variable will *ultimately* be outcome probability, because the response variable used in the computations is not the outcome probability itself. If the probability were modeled directly, some possible combinations of predictor values could lead to probability estimates greater than one or less than zero, and, as we saw earlier, probability by definition can only range between zero and one. To make the math come out right, the probability to be modeled is converted using the logistic or logit transformation to a value that is not zero-one constrained, but can range from minus infinity to infinity – the natural logarithm of the odds. The natural logarithm is equal to 2.7182818, and is often expressed notationally as ln(). The logit transformation is as follows:

**Equation 1.2** $\text{logit}(p) = \ln[p/(1-p)]$

where $p$ = probability. The part of the formula in square brackets should look vaguely familiar. Remember that we were able to convert odds to probability using the formula shown in equation 1.1. In the logistic regression model, we are doing the opposite – converting probability to odds – in order to remove the zero-one constraints, using the following equation:

**Equation 1.3** $o = p/(1-p)$

where $o$ = odds and $p$ = probability. Odds, as we recall, can range from minus infinity to infinity. The logit transformation is just a conversion of probability to the log of the odds. So the dependent variable in a logistic regression equation is the log odds. The form of the logistic regression model, therefore, is:

$$\text{logit}(p) = \alpha + \beta_1 \chi_1 + \beta_2 \chi_2 \ldots \beta_n \chi_n$$

or, more commonly:

$$o = \exp(\alpha + \beta_1 \chi_1 + \beta_2 \chi_2 \ldots \beta_n \chi_n)$$

where $o$ = odds, $\alpha$ is the model intercept term or constant, $\beta_1 - \beta_n$ are the model regression coefficients for risk factor variables 1–$n$, and $\chi_1$–$\chi_n$ are actual values for risk factor variables 1–$n$ that correspond to the model coefficients. If the logit equals the log odds of the model solution (i.e., everything to the right of the equal sign in the logit formula above), then the odds are equal to the exponent (antilog) of the model solution, as in the odds formula above. The exponent of the natural logarithm is usually written exp() or $e^{()}$. Once we have the model we can take the exponent of the regression model solution, which converts log odds to odds, and then convert the odds to probability as in equation 1.1. This way, we can model the simultaneous effects of multiple risk factors on outcome probability, which is what we need to do to make adjustments for the non-independence of predictor variables.

While logistic regression is mainly useful for multivariable work, we should show how the model works in the univariate case just to illustrate the inherent similarity of this method to contingency table methods, and to show how this type of equation is solved. We said above that the most common form of the logistic model is $o = \exp(\alpha + \beta_1\chi_1 + \beta_2\chi_2 \ldots \beta_n\chi_n)$. We put the CHF example data through a logistic model and came up with the following:

$\alpha = -3.4761$

$\beta_1 = 1.2789$

$\chi_1 = 1$ when CHF is present and 0 when CHF is absent

$\beta_n\chi_n$ are ignored because additional variables are not present in the model in this example.

Therefore, odds $= \exp[(-3.4761) + (1.2789 \times \chi_1)]$. When $\chi_1 = 1$ (CHF present):

$$\begin{aligned} \text{odds} &= \exp[(-3.4761) + (1.2789)] \\ &= \exp(-2.1972) \\ &= 0.1111 \end{aligned}$$

the same as at the bottom of Table 1.1 for patients with CHF at the time of surgery. The quantity 1.2789 is retained in the model because the value of the indicator variable for CHF = 1, and $1 \times 1.2789 = 1.2789$. When $\chi_1 = 0$ (CHF absent), the logistic equation simplifies to:

$$\begin{aligned} \text{odds} &= \exp(-3.4761) \\ &= 0.0309 \end{aligned}$$

which is equal to the odds we computed for non-CHF patients. The equation simplifies to the exponent of the intercept term alone because the value of the indicator variable for CHF = 0, and $0 \times 1.2789 = 0$, and $-3.4761 + 0 = -3.4761$. So for CHF present we have odds = 0.1111 and for CHF absent we have 0.0309, as in the contingency table analysis. If we ignore the intercept term and take the exponent of only the regression coefficient for CHF present, exp(1.2789), we get the odds ratio we saw in the contingency table: 3.59. If we wish to convert the odds to probability, we would do so using equation 1.1. For the CHF group it would be $0.1111/(1 + 0.1111) = 0.10$ – ten percent. For the no-CHF group it would be $0.0309/1.0309 = 0.03$ – three percent. We see then that the results of a univariate logistic regression analysis are identical to the results of a contingency table analysis in every respect. We merely need to know how to interpret the regression coefficients to get the correct answers.

The regression coefficients from a multivariable logistic regression model are nothing more than a log-linear combination of risk factor weights that have been mathematically adjusted for one another. We can use the adjusted regression coefficients to compute adjusted odds, and from the odds we can compute an appropriately adjusted risk estimate. We will deal more with the technicalities of the calculations in Chapters 4 and 6, but the concept of multivariate odds computation is essentially the same as the univariate case. In a multivariate model we simply add up a string of variables that have been multiplied by their related regression coefficients. To get a risk estimate for a single patient, the regression coefficients from the model are multiplied by the values of their corresponding variables for that patient, those products are summed, the intercept term is added, and the exponent of the whole thing is taken. This calculation produces the odds of the outcome, which in our example would be hospital death following coronary bypass. Once we have the odds, we divide that quantity by the 1 + odds as in equation 1.1, and get the expected risk. The risk estimate we get at the end of this process is a valid multivariate risk that has been adjusted mathematically for the simultaneous effects of all the variables together. Examples will follow that make the application of this technique clearer in later chapters. Readers who would like to see immediately how the foregoing abstractions are put to use in the multivariable case are referred to Chapter 4 for use of published risk equations, and Chapter 6 for development of new risk equations from a study sample.

Logistic regression has another major advantage beyond its ability to provide adjusted estimates. Models of this type can handle both continuous and dichotomous independent variables. Essentially, data are continuous if they span a continuum. Age, for example, is a continuous variable, because it can be measured not only in whole units (years) but in fractions as well. Children are particularly attuned to this in that they often report their ages as "eight and a half" or "eight and three-quarters". Continuous data can be multiplied through a regression coeffi-

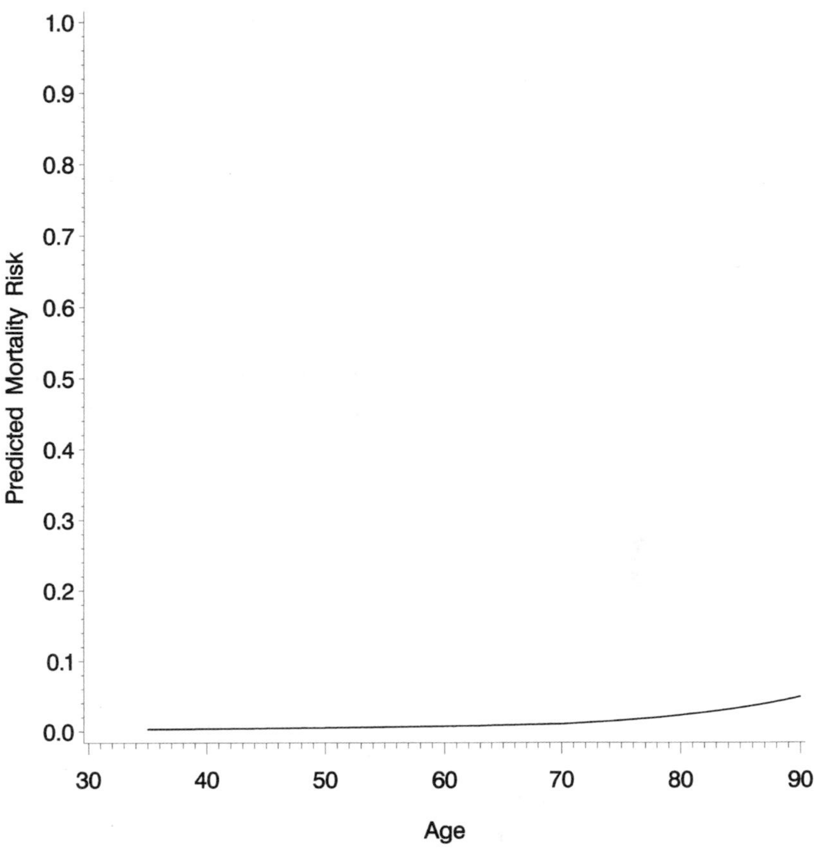


Figure 1.1 Predicted probability by age of in-hospital mortality following coronary bypass surgery.

cient value and estimates along the entire range of the variable can easily be calculated using a computer. The regression coefficient for a continuous variable is interpreted by itself as a change in odds ratio for each unit change in the continuous variable. Likewise, the change in overall probability that is calculated using the regression coefficient, the model intercept and the probability transformation we have already described is change in probability for unit change in age. Figure 1.1 shows the predicted probability of hospital death following coronary bypass surgery taken from the New York State Health Department model (2). This figure was constructed using a logistic regression equation solved for a range of ages. The New York model actually includes 18 variables that combine to predict post-bypass surgery mortality, but in this example we restricted the model to only the variables related to age. It is important to make the point that the age-related coefficients we show here are adjusted for the other variables in the New York model, and that the predictions we are about to make here may not ever actually apply to a patient. For the age variables from this model to be truly appropriate by themselves, the risk we are computing would have to be for a person who was male, had an ejection fraction of 40 percent or greater, and did *not* have any of the following conditions: left main coronary stenosis greater than 90 percent, unstable angina, a myocardial infarction within seven days, a preoperative intra-aortic balloon pump (IABP) device, CHF, an acute myocardial structural defect, acute renal failure, cardiogenic shock, diabetes mellitus, morbid obesity, chronic obstructive pulmonary disease, dialysis dependence, or a previous open heart operation. Many patients who require coronary bypass have at least one of these risk factors, so this is why we say that the following estimate may be unrealistic in that it may never apply to an actual patient's situation.

The New York State model regression coefficient for age is 0.0346. Taking the exponent, exp(0.0346), we see that the odds ratio for postoperative mortality, all other risk factors aside, is 1.0352 per year of age. That is, each year of increasing age adds approximately a 3.5 percent increase in the relative odds. In the New York model, this is only true for patients under 70 years of age. The New York study found that being older than 70 increases risk beyond the simple log-linear term for age that applies to the below-70 age group. Another variable for years beyond the age of 70 becomes non-zero after one reaches 70 and is multiplied by 0.0439 for each year thereafter. So the odds ratio for mortality after bypass surgery for someone over 70 would be $\exp(0.0346 + 0.0439)$ or 1.0817 per year. To get a fixed prediction of the probability of postoperative mortality for a 75 year old, we would use the following equation: $\exp[-6.9605 + (75 \times 0.0346) + (5 \times 0.0439)] = 0.0158$. The probability calculation would be $0.0158/1.0158 = 0.0156$. Expected mortality for a 75 year old with *no other risk factors* would be 1.56 percent.

Figure 1.1 is a plot of the risk predicted from this equation, iterated over a range of ages from 35 to 90 years.

## Selection of variables into logistic models

**Statistical significance**
The probability that an observed statistic was observed by chance.

As we mentioned earlier, risk factors can be useful in sharpening predictions of conditional risk. Technically, this is true when these factors explain variation in predicted probability to a degree that is mathematically separable from the background level of variation. In logistic regression models, variables that account for variance in the outcome over and above that which could be separated from the background by chance alone are said to be *statistically significant.* The technical details of significance testing in logistic models are quite complex, and we will avoid getting into them here. Interested readers are referred to the very good book by Hosmer and Lemeshow (3) for details. The principles of significance testing, though, are simple. In computing risk as we have described it, we are estimating the probability that a discrete event will occur. In our coronary bypass example, the event is death during the period of hospitalization. Ultimately, when the outcome variable is discrete, prediction is a matter of classification. That is, a highly predictive discrete-variable model will predict a death for someone who will actually go on to die, and will predict a survival for someone who actually survives. A statistically significant variable, then, is one that causes the model to do a better job of matching predicted to actual outcomes when the variable is in the model than when it is out. The test that determines whether a risk factor variable improves model classification is known as the likelihood ratio test. "Likelihood", in the generalized mathematical sense, refers to a set of regression parameters that describe the probability that a set of observed data would have occurred as a function of the parameters. As the name suggests, the likelihood ratio significance test is the ratio of model likelihood without the variable to model likelihood with the variable. The likelihood statistic, which is the quantity produced by the likelihood ratio, is evaluated against a chi-square distribution with one degree of freedom to determine the level of statistical significance. For those readers familiar with linear regression analysis, the likelihood ratio is analogous to the model $F$ statistic. For single predictor variable models it assesses the statistical significance of the single predictor. In the multivariable case it describes all of the predictors in the model. In logistic regression, the likelihood ratio test can also be used to evaluate the significance of additional variables being added to a model one at a time or added in groups.

Statistical significance is only one criterion by which variables are evaluated for inclusion in multiple logistic regression models. Other criteria include the biological plausibility of the variable, the proportion of the population at risk in which the variable occurs, and the practicality of ascertaining and measuring the variable under the conditions in which the model will actually be used. We deal with issues of model selection extensively in Chapter 6, and the interested reader is referred to that discussion.

## Model error and classification accuracy

Even the simplest statistical models are associated with a certain amount of error. The sources of error are many, and range from measurement error to general random variation that cannot be pinned down further. Measurement error comes, as its name suggests, from problems with measurement. The values of variables may be measured incorrectly, or the precision (reproducibility) of measurements may be very poor. This can be true of any kind of variable. Errors in measurements of continuous physiological variables such as blood pressure are errors, as much as misclassification of a dichotomous variable such as smoking status would be. Beyond these common sources of "mistake" error, great variation inherently exists in biological systems. Humans are biological creatures, and as such our survival and well-being is governed by many things that are beyond our ability not only to predict, but also to comprehend. If we understood everything that could cause a person to get sick or to die, medical research would be largely unnecessary. Some outcomes simply cannot be predicted beforehand, no matter how good our data. We use the term *model error* as a technical statistical term to indicate variation in outcome that is beyond what a mathematical model can predict. Each regression coefficient is an estimate that has an average value (the coefficient itself), and a measure of the variation associated

**Model error** Variation in outcome beyond what a statistical model can predict.

with that term, which is the standard error. Standard error is related to the more commonly used quantity standard deviation, but it measures the variability in the average that would occur in repeated sampling rather than the variability among the individual observations, as the standard deviation would. An overall estimate of the amount of variance in outcome that the model can account for is known as the coefficient of determination. In linear regression models, the coefficient of determination is called the *R*-square. This is the proportion of the variance in the dependent variable that is explained by the prediction model. Because the computational methods for logistic models are different from those for linear models, the *R*-square cannot be computed in quite the same way for logistic models. However, an analogous quantity that is sometimes called the *R*-square, because of its similar interpretation, is available for logistic regression models. We will not go into the computational details, because they are unnecessary for understanding the meaning of the test. The model coefficient of determination gives us some idea of how predictable an outcome is based on the regression model. A coefficient of determination of 0.10 would indicate that a model explains ten percent of the variance in an outcome. That is not very much explanation, and we should be reluctant to make predictions using a model that accounts for so little variance. On the other hand, a model coefficient of determination of 0.8, 80 percent, would indicate that the model predicts very well, and we could be quite confident making predictions based on such a model. In practice, particularly in biological systems, coefficients of determination of 30–50 percent are about the best we can expect. In general, the sicker the population, the more variable their outcome, so in cases of severe disease we would not expect to have a highly discriminating model. Similarly, when events are rare, we often do not have very strongly predictive models, because so many members of the population have some risk factors but do not experience the outcome.

> ***R*-square**
> Generally, the proportion of all the variance in an outcome that is explained by a statistical model. Also called the coefficient of determination.

Explaining an event such as a death after the fact and predicting it beforehand are entirely different matters. Morbidity and mortality conferences are standard mechanisms for improving quality of care based on retrospective explanation of events. While the results of reviews can be useful for discovering problems in the process of care, the findings of *post hoc* reviews are only useful for risk-stratification projects if they identify risk variables that can be applied prospectively. The goal of risk stratification is to reduce risk over the long term by telling us something about the risk associated with treating patients *before the treatment is begun.* Knowing the risk in advance can help to guide treatment decisions, or maybe even encourage us not to treat at all. In cases where the treatment is as likely to be associated with as bad an outcome as no treatment would be, avoiding treatment altogether might be preferable.

## Generalizing the results

As we saw at the beginning of this chapter, all numerical operations are conducted on sample data, with an eye toward making population inferences. In the majority of risk-stratification situations, hospitals or clinics will be applying published risk formulas – usually logistic regression equations – to their own local data. This involves calculating a risk for each patient by multiplying that patient's data through the logistic equation as described previously, taking the average of the risk for the entire sample, and multiplying the average risk by the number of patients evaluated. The number produced by this calculation is the expected number of events (e.g., coronary bypass hospital deaths) in the local population. The mechanics of applying published logistic equations to local data are described in detail in Chapter 4. For proper application of models – that will lead to generalizable results – attention to the composition of the local sample population as well as that of the study sample on which the equation is based is essential. Ideally, risk estimates will come from good measurements made on unbiased samples. We will cover issues of sample selection and generalizability in detail in Chapters 4, 5 and 6, but as an early concept it is important for readers to understand that logistic regression model predictions are *only as good as the data they are based on.* When using published equations, as most risk-stratification studies do, data from both the original study population and the local population estimates must be of good quality and as close to unbiased as possible. Only good data properly characterized produce accurate statistical models.

## Conclusion

In this chapter we have presented the concepts of sample and population, probability, risk, odds, and use of univariate and multivariate measures of association. Here we have merely laid out the basics, and we will expand on them in greater detail in subsequent chapters. Many of these concepts will still seem vague or mysterious at this point to readers who have not dealt extensively with these issues in the past. Future chapters will revisit each of the concepts we have presented in much greater detail, and will work examples that demonstrate the entire process in practical terms from start to finish, rather than in the necessarily abstract fashion in which we have introduced them here.

## REFERENCES

1 Czeizel AE, Dudas I. Prevention of the first occurrence of neural-tube defects by periconceptional vitamin supplementation. *N Engl J Med* 1992; 327: 1832–5.

2 Hannan EL, Kilburn H, Jr., Racz M, Shields E, Chassin MR. Improving the outcomes of coronary artery bypass surgery in New York State. *JAMA* 1994; 271: 761–6.

3 Hosmer DW, Lemeshow S. *Applied Logistic Regression.* John Wiley & Sons, New York, 1989.

# 2

# Collecting data

In this chapter we will discuss the process and pitfalls of collecting data for risk analysis and stratification. Accurate risk predictions can only be based upon scrupulously collected, high-quality data. Because of the importance of good data as the cornerstone of risk modeling, considerable forethought and effort are warranted in the process of data collection. Many investigators, upon initially pondering a database project, are set upon by an urge to collect (or more likely to arrange for someone else to collect) every remotely relevant data point that comes to mind. We advocate a hearty resistance to this urge, and in fact recommend a deliberate orientation toward collecting as *few* data elements as possible, rather than as many as possible. The goal of data collection and risk modeling should be to identify and collect the smallest amount of data required to provide good prediction and thereby to answer the question at hand. Since this recommendation goes against every investigator's native intellectual curiosity, we provide the following justification.

## Some general comments

Data are expensive and time consuming to collect. This is always true, and shortcuts such as conscripting exhausted residents to collect data or handing out huge blank data collection forms to floor nurses are false economies. Residents rotate on and off service, and have different levels of experience and maturity of judgment, as well as different levels of interest in projects of this type. Surgical residents want to operate, because that is how they accrue credit toward board certification. Running down nursing notes to fill out a database form while the next case is starting will not be a high priority for them, and they will cut corners wherever possible, no matter how much they may fear their Attendings. We, and others who work in the area of risk modeling, have seen this time and time again. Medicine residents need procedures, Family Practice residents need clinic hours, and so on, and all of these people, if given an assignment to collect risk-stratification data, will do just enough of it to prevent them from being fired from their programs. By the time problems with what the house staff have collected are discovered, the residents are on a different service at a hospital on the other side of town. Clinically occupied nurses, likewise, are typically overworked to the point of exasperation, and can be counted on to recite the familiar litany "It's not in my job description" if handed a big research form to fill out. If a project is important enough to do, it is important enough to do well, and doing these things well takes money and personnel who have salary support directly attributable to the project. Anything else leads to problems that will only be discovered late in the process (usually at analysis time) and cannot be fixed easily, or even at all. A clear line of responsibility needs to be established that includes dedicated personnel, and the smallest possible number of people who have the most direct accountability to the project should be involved in collecting and evaluating the data.

Another reason why the study's purpose should be well thought out and the data collected kept to an absolute minimum is that data collection forms tend to be badly controlled if numerous investigators with different interests are involved in the project. Massive data collection forms invented by an ambitious investigator or investigators will almost certainly be mostly blank once they are "completely" filled out. Many data elements conceived early in the database design phase are difficult or impractical to collect. Since a major goal of risk stratification is to summarize the experience of a population, it only makes sense to collect data that will be available for almost everyone in the study sample (not *most* of the sample, which is 51 percent, but *almost all* the sample – more towards 95 percent with a goal of 100 percent). As we will see in Chapter 4, most of the multivariate statistical methods required to do risk analysis throw out incomplete observations (i.e., patients with incomplete data for critical variables), and this is very important. Collecting *any data at all* on patients with incomplete critical variables is throwing money away,

**→ TIP 1**

Only collect data that will be available for nearly all the study sample.

because in the best case all their data are thrown out. In the worst case, "informative missingness" (see Chapter 5) will wipe out entire segments of the study population and bias the conclusions. Critical variables are those that are required to solve a risk model. Two practical guidelines are "don't collect data you're not going to analyze" and "only collect data you're going to analyze on everyone in the population". As suggested by the second of these guidelines, it is preferable not to collect different types of data on different subsets of a population without good justification. Good justification might be when one organ is involved in two or more different procedures. For example, it might be desirable to collect data from all cardiac surgery patients in one database, and to separate the data for valves and for coronaries into separate data tables. Programs such as Microsoft Access allow use of multiple data tables in a single database. Some tables, such as patient information and demographics, could be kept together in one table for all heart patients, so that reports about numbers of heart operations done by year or quarter could be produced with simple queries. However, specific risk and surgical data would need to be linked to sub-tables that would keep the coronary risk data separate from the valve risk data. The key here is that valve patients and coronary bypass patients are kept separate for *analysis* purposes. Different data are required to answer different questions about different populations. Maintaining them in a single database would be a matter of convenience and might improve record keeping, but the separateness of analysis by category of procedure is critical and should not be violated.

> **➔ TIP 2**
>
> Don't collect data you're not going to analyze. If you don't know how you will use it right now, don't collect it.

As an extension of this concept, it is never acceptable to collect different data for different patients undergoing the *same* treatment if this difference in data collected is based at all on the risk factor profile, severity of illness, etc. For example, it would not be appropriate to collect ejection fraction data on all patients who had cardiac catheterizations in the local hospital but to ignore ejection fraction data on all patients who came into hospital having been catheterized elsewhere because the films were hard to get. In a referral center, this could introduce a massive bias because patients who come in with catheterization studies from another institution and do not have them repeated locally might be critically ill ambulance transfers who community medical centers did not feel qualified to manage. Differential data collection based on risk factors or on other things that influence risk factors can have disastrous effects on the validity of conclusions made from risk models. All these things must be considered before beginning a risk-stratification-related data collection project. As with the other hazards we have mentioned, many of these problems can be minimized through the use of a focused research question set up in advance. The first stage in deciding what to collect is deciding how that data will be analyzed. Deciding what to analyze depends on the question to be answered.

## Identifying a question

Hopefully, no one would undertake a risk-stratification project without some sort of question in mind. However, in our experience assisting others with projects of this type, the initial questions are not always well thought through. It should be borne in mind that risk-stratification studies are intended to be primarily standardization studies. Their main goal is to provide some sort of appropriate benchmark against which to compare local data involving a particular disease or treatment–disease combination. For example, use of risk stratification to compare a medical center's in-hospital mortality data following a coronary bypass operation to a recognized national standard is an appropriate use. It would be substantially less appropriate to use a risk-stratification project to study the adoption of a new treatment, say a minimally invasive coronary bypass operation, to determine whether the minimally invasive procedure is better than open surgery, using only an open-surgery standard from the literature as a comparison. Comparison studies rightfully require local, contemporaneous comparison groups, and optimally are done as randomized clinical trials.

Using published data that arise from a different population than the one currently under study is asking for trouble. For example, it is possible to imagine a minimally invasive coronary surgery program applying their patient data to a risk model for open coronary surgery. Suppose that the risk-stratified results indicated that the minimally invasive surgery had lower mortality than would have been expected for open surgery. Would that show that minimally invasive coronary surgery was better than open coronary surgery? Certainly, the temptation would be to claim that the local minimally invasive population has been standardized to the published open-surgery population on the basis of risk factors, and that the results were directly interpretable because of the standardization. In fact, the study would have been undertaken in the first place to justify exactly this claim. But if the populations studied were not materially comparable, other explanations may, and probably would, exist. Minimally invasive techniques for coronary surgery vary widely in their scope and approach. Some use a conventional sternotomy approach with a smaller incision but with all the usual instrumentation. Others modify the technique more, by using a balloon to occlude the aorta intravascularly rather than by using an external clamp. Some centers do minimally invasive coronary surgery only in younger patients with limited disease to achieve improved cosmetic results. Other centers consider minimally invasive techniques to be less physiologically demanding, and use them only on patients for whom the open-chest approach is considered too risky. Each of these hypothetical populations is highly selected relative to the general population with coronary heart disease, who make up the open-chest risk-stratification population. Differences in the population cause problems with interpretation of the results, as we will see in more detail in Chapter 5. Risk populations must be comparable in order for the estimates to be useful, and population comparability is a major factor in shaping the research question. It is the question to be answered, ultimately, which determines the data to be collected and the choice of risk model.

> **➔ TIP 3**
> Allow the research question to determine the choice of risk model.

When comparing local data to risk data that are already published, much of the form of the question will depend on what question was asked in the original study. The research question of the local study will need to match that of the reference study as closely as possible. In the case of mortality following coronary bypass surgery using the New York State model as a reference, for example, the research question would be "what is the risk-adjusted in-hospital mortality in our local population following coronary bypass surgery?". This is different from "what is the 30-day mortality following coronary artery bypass surgery?", and "what is the intra-operative coronary bypass mortality?". Since most coronary bypass patients are discharged from the hospital within a week following surgery, and some patients presumably die after they go home, we would expect hospital mortality to underestimate 30-day mortality. By the same token, since most coronary bypass patients who die in hospital do so during recovery, we would expect hospital mortality to overestimate intraoperative (i.e., on the operating table) deaths. For the study question regarding our local data to give us estimates that are directly comparable to the New York study, we would need to measure the outcome over the same post-bypass period as the New York study did (i.e., the period of post-bypass hospitalization). Once an appropriate study question has been identified, it is time to move on to considering data collection.

## Identification of variables

For risk-stratification studies that are based on published risk equations, identification of the variables necessary to solve the equations is straightforward. The paper in which the equations are published will list the variables and will give some description of what they represent and how they were ascertained. Most variables that are contained in multiple logistic regression risk studies will usually be indicator variables. Indicator variables are variables that have the value 1 when a risk factor is present, and 0 (with some exceptions as we will see later) when the risk factor is absent. Making indicator variables requires a variable definition of some kind. An indicator variable for diabetes mellitus, for example, might be 1 when a person is insulin dependent, and 0 otherwise. Alternatively, it might be 1 whenever a person takes any kind of regular medication for their diabetes mellitus and 0 otherwise. Good studies will give details of how the variables are ascertained and what the criteria are for classification. Poor instructions for classification on the part of the source article or poor adherence to the classification system on the part of the investigative team leads to improper risk factor classification. Poor classification leads to some people with the risk factor being classified as not having it, or some people without the risk factor being classified as having it. Either way, the estimates of the local population will be biased by the misclassification. If misclassification is random (i.e., it does not go in only one direction), the effect will be mainly to reduce the magnitude of the association and consequently the statistical power of the estimates.

If the bias is in one direction, with most misclassification going, for example, toward a 0 coding (risk factor absent) rather than toward 1 (risk factor present), then the resulting estimates of probability will be biased in one direction as well. If a risk factor is frequently missed in a local population, the risk estimate based on a standard equation will be lower than it should have been. If a risk factor is frequently coded as present when it is really absent, the risk estimate for the local population will be too high (both of these illustrations assume that the risk factor is a harmful, rather than a protective one, by the way). It is extremely important that variable definitions be followed closely and that ascertainment of the status of each of the variables is as accurate as possible.

Besides the variables required to solve a risk equation, individual centers may be interested in collecting *some* additional variables for future research. As long as the previous warnings about not overdoing the data capture are heeded, collection of a few extra data points is a reasonable thing to do. The variables should be related to the outcome, to other variables, or to both in some biologically plausible way and plans should exist for how the variables would be used and interpreted in the future. Neither fishing expeditions nor data that are not analyzed are worth the time it takes to fool with them. Figure 2.1 shows the data collection form we use to collect data on clean coronary bypasses for risk stratification at our institution. The variables required to solve several widely used coronary bypass risk-stratification equations are included, as well as some other data we are collecting for other reasons.

## Case definition

**Case**
An instance of the event or outcome being studied.

**Non-case**
A *confirmed* non-event.

As with risk factor variables, a definition of what constitutes a *case* of the outcome needs to be established as well. Again, as with the predictor variables, the definition of the outcome variable is most easily obtained in studies based on published models that give a detailed description of how a case is defined. We use the technical term "case definition" to denote the criteria by which an outcome event is said to have occurred. Case definition also refers to the procedure for determining that a patient is not a "case". When more than two outcomes are possible, defining a *non-case* is as important as defining a case. Because the outcome variable affects the interpretation of *all* the risk factor variables, case definition is one of the most important topics in the area of data collection and management. Where risk is to be compared to a published standard, cases should be defined exactly as they are in the reference population. For hard endpoints such as mortality, the definition is straightforward, although even for hard endpoints such as this, the time frame within which it occurs is part of the case definition. The case definition is shaped largely by the research question as we saw above. In cases where the endpoint is less clear-cut, such as a pathological diagnosis, a quality of life measure, or some other measure that requires professional judgment or administration of some sort of psychometric instrument, attention to the training of the evaluating personnel is critical. In some cases where endpoints show particularly large variation, a formal process of training, testing, and certification may be required. Some measure of reliability should be employed in the training process and should be applied to collected data periodically as a quality control procedure. Reliability can be technically complicated to measure, so a qualified statistician should be consulted for advice on the design and analysis of reliability studies.

**→ TIP 4**

Be aware of sources of competing risks, which can bias results.

Competing risks may also affect case definition. It is often true that patients can be removed from the risk of a study endpoint by something other than the successful completion of a study time period. For example, if we were interested in studying the probability of major stroke following coronary artery bypass surgery, we would need to consider all other occurrences that might interfere with the determination that a stroke had or had not occurred. Patients who die intraoperatively, for example, do not recover from the anesthetic and cannot be evaluated clinically for postoperative stroke. A person who died without awakening should not be reported as a non-stroke, because we do not know whether a stroke occurred in that person or not. If a significant rate of operative mortality were to occur, and the rate of stroke were high in the population as well, a large bias in the reported estimate of stroke would occur if the operative deaths were coded as non-strokes. Consider the following hypothetical example. Suppose that a new operation was developed for a certain cardiac problem and we wanted to determine whether it had an acceptable risk-adjusted morbidity and mortality.

Figure 2.1 (*opposite*) Sample form used to collect data for coronary bypasses at our institutions. Captures the basic variables of interest to us as well as all the data necessary to solve the New York State model. This form is actually the data entry screen for a Microsoft Access database. Preoperative variables used to solve the New York State and Cleveland Clinic risk models (only preoperative data are acceptable here).

*# Dz vessels*, number of diseased coronary arteries; *# Previous heart ops*, number of previous open heart operations; *Acute structural defect*, cardiac acute structural defect, ventricular rupture, ventricular tumor, large necrotic area, etc.; *Anatomy unknown*, data on extent of coronary disease unavailable from the chart; *Aortic and mitral valve Dz*, untreated valve disease (a repaired or replaced valve is not classified as diseased as long as it is competent); *Cardiomegaly*, clinical finding of cardiomegaly; *Cerebrovasc Dz*, clinical cerebrovascular disease; *CHF*, clinically apparent congestive heart failure; *Chronic R.I.*, clinical chronic renal insufficiency (serum creatinine persistently >1.5 mmol/24 hours); *Complications*, text field for any unusual findings or complications that may be helpful for future studies; *COPD*, clinical diagnosis of chronic obstructive pulmonary disease; *Creat*, serum creatinine in mmol/l; *CVA*, documented cerebrovascular accident; *Diabetes*, diabetes mellitus (type 1 or 2) requiring therapy; *Dialysis dependent*, patient requires dialysis to maintain creatinine (florid renal failure); *Done*, data entry operator's indication that the record is complete; *EF*, left ventricular ejection fraction by radionuclide gated ventriculography, cardiac catheterization or echocardiographic estimation; *Encounter*, hospital identification number for a particular episode of care; *Entry*, data entry operator's identification and date of record completion; *Hct*, hematocrit; *Hypertension*, diastolic blood pressure >95 mmHg; *IV inotropes*, intravenous inotropic agents required to maintain blood pressure; *IV nitrates*, intravenous nitrates required to control angina or blood pressure; *LM stenosis*, left main coronary artery stenosis; *Mitral regurg*, clinical signs of mitral valve regurgitation; *Most recent MI*, most recent myocardial infarction; *On COPD Meds*, evidence from the medical chart that the patient is on chronic COPD therapy; *Pack years*, packs of cigarettes smoked per day times number of years smoked; *Preop IABP*, preoperative requirement for intra-aortic balloon pump counterpulsation; *Prior Smk*, prior smoking history; *Prior vasc surg*, previous vascular surgery for atherosclerosis (trauma would not count); *PTCA emergency*, emergency operation due to percutaneous transluminal coronary angioplasty or other cardiac catheterization laboratory misadventure (coronary artery rupture, dissection, etc.); *Renal failure*, serum creatinine >1.9 mmol/l or dialysis dependence; *Severe LV dysfunction*, severe clinical ventricular hypokinesis; *Ventric aneurysm*, cardiac ventricular aneurysm.

**OUTCOMES NYH DATABASE**

Encounter: 1

Date surg:

Surgeon

Current smoking: ○ Yes ◉ No ○ Unkn

Prior smk: ◉ Yes ◉ No ○ Unkn

Height: 0 inches

Weight: 0 lbs

Creat: 0

Hct: 0

Pack years: 0

| | Yes | No | Unkn |
|---|---|---|---|
| CHF | ○ | ◉ | ○ |
| Renal failure | ○ | ◉ | ○ |
| Chronic R.I. | ○ | ◉ | ○ |
| Hypertension | ○ | ◉ | ○ |
| Diabetes | ○ | ◉ | ○ |
| COPD | ○ | ◉ | ○ |
| On COPD meds | ○ | ◉ | ○ |
| Cardiomegaly | ○ | ◉ | ○ |

| | Yes | No | Unkn |
|---|---|---|---|
| Aortic valve Dz | ○ | ◉ | ○ |
| Mitral valve Dz | ○ | ◉ | ○ |
| Mitral regurg | ○ | ◉ | ○ |
| Other valve Dz | ○ | ◉ | ○ |
| Cerebrovasc Dz | ○ | ◉ | ○ |
| CVA | ○ | ◉ | ○ |
| Ventric aneurysm | ○ | ◉ | ○ |
| Prior vasc surg | ○ | ◉ | ○ |

Angina: ○ Unstable ◉ Stable ○ None ○ Unknown

Most recent MI: ○ <6 hours ○ <24 hours ○ 1–7 days ○ 8–21 days ○ >22 days ◉ none

# Dz vessels: 0

LM stenosis >90 ○

LM stenosis >50 ○

Anatomy unknown ○

Click for Yes

| | |
|---|---|
| Cardiogenic shock | ○ |
| Acute structural defect | ○ |
| Preop IABP | ○ |
| IV nitrates | ○ |
| IV inotropes | ○ |
| PTCA emergency | ○ |
| Severe LV dysfunction | ○ |
| Dialysis dependent | ○ |

Operative priority: ○ unknown ◉ elective ○ urgent ○ emergent

EF: 0

# Previous heart ops: 0

Done ○

Entry: John 9/27/99

Complications:

Suppose that the standard stroke rate following the usual procedure for this problem was seven percent. Now suppose that the true postoperative stroke rate for the new operation was ten percent. Suppose further that the intraoperative mortality for the new operation was 30 percent. Now consider a population of 100 patients. If 30 percent (30 patients of 100) of the population died before they could be evaluated for stroke, the true stroke rate, still ten percent as we've assumed, will be seven strokes in 70 evaluable patients (7/70 = 10%). Seventy are evaluable because 30 of the 100 were removed from risk by death, and 70 remained at risk of a stroke. If, however, the 30 that died were *not* removed from risk in the database but instead were improperly listed as non-strokes during data analysis, the stroke rate that would be estimated using the database would be 7/100. That is, seven strokes observed over the 70 at risk plus the 30 no longer at risk that were improperly classified as non-strokes. This classification error would lead to an estimated seven percent stroke rate and the incorrect conclusion that the new procedure had the same stroke rate as the old. When a competing risk removes a patient from the risk of a primary endpoint, the variable that denotes the primary outcome should be coded as missing rather than as 0 or outcome-absent. This is extremely important.

## Case ascertainment

Case ascertainment is related to case definition. Once the case definition is determined, some effort is required to determine that all cases and relevant non-cases that exist in a particular target population are available for sample. This is not to say that all members of a target population *have* to be sampled, only that they need to be *available* for sampling in an unbiased way. Many systematic impediments to sampling particular segments of the population may exist, and these need to be identified so that a truly representative sample of cases can be ascertained. For example, if a group of asthma patients were being followed for Emergency Room utilization and only local hospital admission records were used in case ascertainment, some of the most severe cases might go unreported when patients were too sick to make it to that particular hospital.

**➔ TIP 5**

Complete case ascertainment is essential for reliable estimates.

Although the outcome variable biases are the ones that give the greatest concern, risk factor biases can be very misleading as well. An investigator who wanted to study the effects of alcohol consumption on recurrent coronary disease in older adults might find that older patients who consume more alcohol have very low rates of reoperation for coronary artery disease. This would be a useful finding, unless it were true that many heavy drinkers suffered fatal heart attacks and did not need to come back for repeat bypasses. Subtle effects that remove people from risk *before they would come to the attention of investigators* are known as harvesting effects, and are very difficult to pin down and identify completely. These are different from the competing risk problems on-study that we mentioned previously, where proper classification can be obtained by good follow-up.

## Planning data collection

As we have seen, many theoretical issues including sources of bias, variable definitions, and case ascertainment need to be considered in any plan for data collection. But the matters of where, when and how data will be collected are also important, and some practical issues related to what we might call the ergonomics of data collection should be considered. Where will data come from? In what order or time sequence will the data values be encountered during data collection? How soon after the end of the observation period will data become available? Where will data be recorded in the time interval between treatment, outcome and data entry for the study? Will any data not captured immediately be lost? If so, how will data that arise outside of normal working hours be identified and captured? Asking simple questions such as these during the process of designing the data collection forms can go a long way toward reducing the difficulty of data collection later on. If, for example, chart review will be the primary means of data collection, simple things like paying attention to the order of chart flow can have large effects on the amount of time and effort that are involved in abstracting. For example, if demographics are the first things that appear in the chart, the area for collecting demographic information should be at the beginning

**➔ TIP 6**

Organize data collection forms in a way that follows the natural flow of data from the source documents.

of the data collection form as well. If a dozen variables can be retrieved from the anesthesia record in a surgical study, those variables should be in the same area of the data collection form. If data are being entered directly into computers, variables collected in the same place should be on the same data entry screen. Any small change in data collection form layout that reduces chart flipping, form page shuffling or computer scrolling will have an enormous cumulative effect on abstractor time and aggravation over several thousand records reviewed.

As notebook computers become smaller, lighter and are powered by longer-life batteries, the temptation to go paperless in the collection of data becomes stronger. Using paper forms to collect data that are going to be entered into the computer eventually anyway can be awkward and resource consuming. It is often necessary in the case of larger paper-form-based projects for some people to collect data and some people to enter data, and that may be a costly redundancy. In our view, the decision of whether or not to do a paperless study depends mainly on the source of data and the extent of the requirement for source documentation. Our groups have both paper-trail and paperless studies in progress at the present. Studies that are based entirely on data that are recorded in hospital charts can be completely paperless. The charts themselves can serve as source documents if an audit trail is required. Where source documents are not available (e.g., a value has to be read off a monitor in the intensive care unit or the operating room), some sort of record that substantiates the data recorded in the computer should be available. Many studies that are externally sponsored or that are subject to regulatory oversight are required to have a paper component with a clear line of supporting source documentation.

Assignment of responsibility for case ascertainment, and for data collection, management and analysis is an integral part of study planning. A clear line of accountability needs to be established, and each person, from data collector to investigator, needs to be properly trained in his or her job, and needs to express an appropriate level of understanding of, and buy in to, the project. Periodic status reporting for each phase of the project is appropriate, as are regular (weekly to annually depending on the age of the study and the smoothness with which it has been running) meetings of the full team. The full team means everybody from the principal investigator to the part-time data entry operator. The people closest to the data will almost always have the best impressions of how things are going.

## Selecting data collection software

The determination of what software to use is based mainly on the scope of the project, but it is also based on the skills and preferences of the person or persons who will be responsible for using it. An elaborate structured query language database such as Oracle or Microsoft Access is probably overkill for a project that requires ten variables. A spreadsheet program is usually more than adequate for small projects, and most spreadsheets can be programmed to solve equations necessary for risk calculations as well. Spreadsheet programs are also more likely to be familiar to office personnel or others without advanced computer skills.

> **➔ TIP 7**
> Simple spreadsheet programs are often acceptable for small projects. Don't overdo the data collection process.

For larger projects, particularly those that require linking of data records across multiple tables or where a standardized report format is desirable, relational database products are usually preferable. Database programs have the further significant advantage of allowing data to be entered on forms specially designed for the project, and they can be programmed to provide a certain level of validity enhancement, such as field cross-checking, double data entry, and so on. They can also warn when critical variables are missing, and hold a data record open (i.e., register it as "incomplete") when critical variables are missing. Many databases can also be password protected, which may be important for reasons of data security and patient confidentiality. Password assignment also allows for determination of which operator entered which data, and this can be useful for auditing and for providing feedback to operators on data entry accuracy and the like.

In cases where data collection will be paperless, the database should be able to record the time and date of each entry, when it was last modified, and the identities of any data system operators that have entered or edited data. This information is very helpful for auditing, especially when unusual or implausible observations are recorded, and can also be helpful for legal reasons having to do with scientific integrity and clinical results.

## Data entry

Data entry procedures depend on the number of variables to be captured, the intensity with which data will need to be scrutinized for accuracy, and several other considerations, such as whether some data from other sources can be read in electronically. For informal studies with small numbers of variables, hand-keyed data entry into a spreadsheet program is usually acceptable. For sponsored studies (pharmaceutical or device studies supported by the manufacturers, government-funded studies, etc.), full function databases that use double data entry and field range and logic checks are the standard. Double data entry requires each data field to be keyed twice. The program compares the two entries, and if they match it writes them to the record. If not, the program will prompt the operator to re-enter the data, and will continue until two matching entries are observed. Some databases can be programmed to keep statistics on the number of non-matching entries and can report error rates. Error rate reporting can be useful not only for measuring operator skill and guiding training efforts, but can also help to identify data that are chronically difficult to enter. Difficult data formats can often be simplified to improve the accuracy of data entry and make life easier for the operators.

**→ TIP 8**

Large studies will often be too complex for spreadsheet data collection. Database products contain many useful tools that can improve the speed and accuracy of data entry. Use them.

Use of pick-lists, dialog boxes and the like can also speed data entry dramatically and improve accuracy. These data entry tools provide lists of potential entries or click boxes that save keystrokes. They also limit the range of entries that can be made and thereby reduce the likelihood of data entry error. If, for example, a three-physician group, Drs Smith, Jones and Howard, were collecting data on a group of their patients, a variable for which doctor did the treatment would be desirable. But typing in the names for each entry would be time consuming and the potential for error would be great. Misspellings, typographical errors, etc., that were accidentally recorded to the database would attribute patients to doctors who did not exist, and the summary statistics for the three actual doctors would be incorrect. With a pick-list, the operator simply pulls down a menu and clicks on the appropriate doctor. Typographical errors and misspellings are eliminated, because the opportunity to make such errors does not exist with a pick-list.

In addition to using such automated shortcuts, it is often possible to download certain data elements from other sources. Electronic transfer reduces errors and reduces redundant work, provided it is done appropriately. For example, at our institution, the hospital identification number is used to track all patients' records. We use the hospital's billing system to identify coronary bypass cases that meet our criteria, and then use the hospital identification number combined with an admission date identifier as the primary key in our Microsoft Access database to give each patient a unique identifier for a particular encounter. Rather than have our data entry operators type in a 15-digit number every time (and risk making transcription errors), we capture the encounter numbers directly from the billing system and download it into our risk database. This is an example of an appropriate use of electronic data transfer.

Many times, however, possible electronic transfers that seem like a good idea turn out not to work very well. We worked recently with someone who wanted to download blood pressure and oxygen saturation data from intensive care unit monitors directly into a database. The problem was that this person wanted to capture only one average value each day, and the monitoring devices did not have the ability to average and report the data. We could have dealt with this easily enough by writing a separate program that would take the data off the intensive care unit system and average them, but many sources of artifact are present in such systems, and automated methods for sorting them out are not good. If a patient rolls over on an ear oximeter probe or kinks a radial artery catheter, streamed monitor data can be inaccurate for hours, and can cause bad things to happen to the averages. Our view is that electronic data transfers into risk databases should only be done for variables that have previously been reviewed and verified in their original sources. Otherwise, the likelihood of measurement error is high and this error may cause problems for the power and interpretability of the results.

## Pilot testing

Data collection forms usually undergo a certain amount of modification once they are put to use. As differences between the way data are actually collected and the way data collection was planned become apparent, some changes that will improve the process are usually warranted. It is extremely desirable to identify problems and make changes as early in the process as possible, and ideally to do it before data collected on new forms are actually important. That is, pilot studies of data collection should be done if at all possible before new forms are used to collect important data. A brief analysis should be undertaken using pilot data as well, to make sure that the data being collected can be used to answer the research question in the way that was intended in the research design. One of the problems with collecting important data using untried data collection forms is that databases are difficult to revise partway through a project. If, for example, a decision is made midway through a project to collect an additional risk factor variable that had not been collected previously, the ability to use the new variable will be restricted only to the population that follows implementation of the new process. If we have 1000 patients in a cardiac surgery database and we decide at the halfway point that family history of coronary disease is important, we will only be able to examine its effect in the second half of the patient group. No data will be available on the first half of the study cohort. Big changes in the protocol partway through cause major problems for interpretation and the generalizability of estimates, and should be avoided if at all possible. Pilot testing of data forms and analyses can be very valuable for making sure that the data collection that is planned will lead to the proper assessment of the research question down the road.

**➔ TIP 9**

Pilot testing a data collection form can save a great deal of trouble down the road.

## Quality control

Some program for quality control should be designed at the time the study is planned. We mentioned previously that several database-related techniques can be used, such as double data entry, range checks, logic checks, etc. Range checks allow the database programmer to limit the range of possible entries. In a study of an adult cardiac surgery population, for example, a criterion could be set for patient height that would issue a warning whenever a value of less than 4 feet or more than 7 feet was entered. Logic checks compare the value of certain data fields against others. If, for example, a field that asked if a patient had ever smoked were entered as “no”, the next question in the sequence about how many packs per day were smoked could be suppressed. Automated techniques are the first line of defense against data entry and coding errors.

Not all errors can be avoided using such techniques, however. Incorrect entries may result from the transcription of poor handwriting, misread values from patient records, etc., and these may fall within physiological ranges that would not be detected by automated program checks. Also, some of the job of classification often falls to the person who is collecting the data. In chart review series, for example, a judgment about whether a patient had unstable angina on admission to hospital may need to be inferred from the chart even when explicit statements about the type of angina are not made. Patients admitted for coronary bypass through the Emergency Room who were receiving intravenous nitrates are likely to have had unstable angina. It is possible (indeed, essential) to develop standards as part of the process of defining the variable and case. Still, some variability in how much of the chart is reviewed and how deeply the abstractor will dig to meet the case criteria will always be present. It will vary between chart abstractors, it will vary within an individual abstractor over time, and may even vary day by day, depending on whether five or 50 charts are reviewed at a single sitting. For this reason, periodic reliability studies are desirable, to examine person-to-person variability (known as inter-rater reliability) and variability within each person (known as intra-rater reliability). Large differences in either dimension are grounds for additional training, and may signal a need for greater simplification or standardization of the case definition criteria. Large amounts of intra-rater variability may indicate overworking of the abstractors as well. The best reliability studies of these types are done using repeated sampling and random-effects analysis of variance models. A qualified statistician should be involved in the design and analysis of any reliability studies, as these studies are actually quite complex.

Random audits on segments of the population are useful for quality control and for identifying data that are difficult to categorize. Depending on the size of the study sample, random audits of one to ten percent are usually recommended. Ideally, a computerized random-number-generator process should identify records selected for random audits. Other "random" techniques are not desirable because they are not actually very random in the statistical sense. The purpose of any randomization process is to ensure that each member of a population has an equal probability of being selected, because equality of probability is what provides the least chance of bias in accumulating samples. Things like month of birth, odd day/even day at clinic, etc., have all been shown to produce non-random (i.e., biased) results.

## Source documentation

Source documentation or backup documentation refers to a set of documents that show the original source of the data entered into the computer. The most common source documents for medical risk-stratification studies are medical charts. Ideally, every variable that exists in a computer database will be drawn from an identifiable place in a medical chart. Most sponsored studies, and all studies that are subject to the overview of governmental regulatory agencies, are required to maintain source documents, usually for a period of seven years after the conclusion of the study. Source documentation provides an audit trail and adds another facet to the accuracy enhancement provided by programmable database techniques. It also provides backup information in the event that the integrity of the database is ever questioned. Although we have said that informal local studies can be done paperless, when there is any doubt, it is best to keep source documents.

**→ TIP 10**

When in doubt, keep source documents.

## Regulatory issues

Requirements for institutional review board (IRB) approval for risk-stratification studies vary by institution and project type. Local IRB offices can provide institution-specific guidelines, and it is always a good idea to check with the IRB before starting any form of data collection. Confidentiality of patient data, on the other hand, is a legal requirement under any circumstances, and must be maintained whether local IRB rules require the project to be reviewed or not. Confidentiality of medical records has been a hot topic with the United States Congress in the last few years, and institutional legal departments can be instrumental in helping investigators stay abreast of shifting regulations. We recommend that investigators establish a relationship with their legal departments, because legal compliance is an increasingly important part of medical research. Generally, information that could be used to identify individual patients must be removed from reports or coded in such a way that it is unrecognizable. Source data or copies of sensitive information should be kept in locked files. Locked offices, computer password protection or both should be used to control access to data.

## Conclusion

Data collection is a central component of the risk-stratification process and as such deserves careful consideration and planning. Accurate predictions of risk can be obtained only with high-quality data that are appropriate to the research question. Studies should be designed with a specific question in mind, and care should be taken in the design phase to minimize opportunities for misclassification and missing-data problems to arise. Definitions of formal cases and predictor variables should be set out in advance, and a plan for complete ascertainment of cases and non-cases should be made. For larger or more detailed projects, database programs that can provide assistance in accuracy enhancement and automation of repetitive tasks should be used wherever possible. Source documentation should be available in most cases for quality control and audit purposes, and proper care should be taken to ensure that regulatory and confidentiality requirements are met.

possible, it is best to use studies that were designed for use as risk analysis studies in the production of local risk expectations. These studies will have been produced from series of consecutive patients that meet the case/non-case definition, rather than from the highly selected populations that might have been assembled from cohort or clinical trial studies, and will be more heterogeneous and therefore applicable to the clinical milieu. Clinical research studies, and clinical trials in particular, usually follow long protocols that look only at very highly selected groups of patients. In order for a randomized treatment protocol to be conducted ethically, *all* patients enrolled must be eligible to receive *any* of the treatments being studied. What this means in terms of patient inclusion/exclusion rules is that only patients who can receive any of the study treatments can be admitted. This leads to very narrow criteria for inclusion, in which all patients must be "ideal" candidates. In the real world of clinical practice, on the other hand, many treatments will be administered to patients who are less than "ideal", because the range of people who have certain diseases that require treatment is broad, and some people will have multiple problems. However, when there are no risk studies in a particular clinical area, cohort and clinical trial studies can be used instead if they meet a few important criteria in addition to those that pertain to risk studies. Not much has been written about the design of dedicated risk-stratification studies and their strengths and weaknesses. In general, because risk-stratification studies have conceptual similarities to efficacy-oriented clinical research studies, the strengths and weaknesses of the standard clinical research designs are applicable to risk studies as well. The designs we review below are mainly from the efficacy-orientated clinical research literature, but their inferential approach is conceptually analogous to that of risk stratification. The only real difference is that risk stratification focuses on differences between populations that are treated the same, rather than differences between groups of patients who are treated differently. Risk-stratification studies do indeed share some fundamental assumptions with other types of clinical research studies; for example, the assumption that all patients in the study share a common indication for a treatment is a major one.

**→ TIP 2**

Risk stratification measures differences in outcome between populations that are treated the same. Efficacy research measures differences in outcome between groups of patients that are treated differently.

The quality of studies that have been published in the clinical research literature varies quite a bit. For risk stratification, a published study is

**Table 3.1** Hierarchy of clinical evidence

1. Randomized controlled trials
2. Prospective cohort studies
3. Case–control studies
4. Cross-sectional studies
5. Case reports/Case series
6. Expert opinion

used as a reference that serves as the standard by which local results are judged, so the quality of the reference study can have a great deal of bearing on the conclusions of a risk-stratification study. The strength of the research design, the size of the sample, the attention paid by the original researchers to bias and other possible problems, the quality of the hypothesis tests, and the appropriateness of the statistical analysis all contribute to the overall quality of a published study. Many types of study design exist, and each has strengths and weaknesses.

If a variety of studies have been published on a particular topic, the choice of which one to use as a standard, assuming that they are otherwise of comparable quality, will depend more on the study design than anything else. Table 3.1 shows a hierarchy of study designs arranged according to inferential strength. Unlike risk-stratification studies, the designs that follow were originally developed to answer questions about specific treatments, exposures or other risk factors. The control for "confounding" variables offered by each design technique was developed in order to allow for measurement of the independent contribution of the main variable of interest to the outcome. In risk-stratification studies, no *a priori* hierarchy exists among the risk factors being studied. The object of risk stratification is to determine how multiple risk factors work together to modify the risk of an outcome. Despite the differences in focus, risk-stratification studies arise from the background of other research designs, and the strengths and weaknesses of the designs are as pertinent to overall risk assessments as they are to single treatments or exposures.

## Classical clinical research

By classic clinical research, we mean clinical experiments and epidemiological studies. Randomized, controlled clinical trials are generally held by the scientific community to be the gold standard in any evaluation of the effects of a medical intervention. Randomized trials always study some sort of treatment, because the term "randomized" means that treatments are allocated to trial participants on a random basis. The rationale for random treatment allocation is that a treatment administered randomly is not based on any characteristic of the patient. Each patient who enters the trial has a known probability of being assigned to any treatment. Usually, the probability is equal – half the patients receive the investigational treatment and half receive a control treatment (such as a placebo). Some trials use randomization schemes that alter the treatment ratio to an allocation that is not 1:1. We were recently involved in a study of lung volume reduction surgery in which half the patients in our center were assigned to surgery and half to medical therapy, but among the surgical group another randomization allocated patients to open-chest versus thoracoscopic resection. Although it may seem counter to medical judgment to allocate treatment in a way that is unrelated to the patient's condition or any other characteristic, this is actually the best way to sort out the independent effects of the treatment. In order to qualify for a clinical trial, all patients have to be eligible to receive any of the possible treatments. It is only *within a group of eligible patients* that randomized treatment allocation is used. A major virtue of the randomized design is that, by providing treatment that is unrelated to, and therefore not biased by, patient condition, patient condition variables are separated from the effect of treatment. The randomization process tends to even out differences between clinical variables among the treatment groups, so that in well-designed studies the groups are almost always comparable. Another major virtue of randomization is that it controls automatically for potentially confounding variables that may interfere with the interpretation of the results. This research design has the further advantage of being able to control for confounding variables that either did not occur to the investigators or were unknown at the beginning of the study. Randomized selection of patients to treatment is completely separated from *all* patient characteristics; even those we do not know about or cannot measure. The widely publicized example of fenfluramine-phentermine (fen-phen) heart-valve disease provides a good example. A randomized clinical trial of two formulations of dexfenfluramine (a commonly prescribed isomer of the "fen" in fen-phen) versus placebo was begun in order to assess the effects of the drugs on weight loss between the two groups of obese subjects (1). At the time the clinical trial was started, nothing had been published about the possible association of the fenfluramines with heart-valve disease. The valve-disease story broke in the first year of the clinical trial, and the trial was stopped because it was not considered ethical to continue to expose study participants to a potentially hazardous treatment. At the time the controversy came to light, many questions about confounding between obesity and heart-valve disease were raised, and the question of whether it was the fenfluramine itself or other things that might cause people to seek fenfluramine treatment was left open. Because data from the clinical trial were available, the patients could be brought in and evaluated for valve disease by echocardiography, and a comparison between the treated and the untreated patient groups could be undertaken. Trial data were already blinded and placebo-controlled, so a very good design for evaluating valvulopathy was created without the investigators having intended to start such a study at the beginning.

As it turned out, the dexfenfluramine-treated patients did have a higher prevalence of valvular disease at the end of the study than the placebo-treated patients. Although baseline measurements of valve function were not made, the randomized design makes it extremely likely that the groups were balanced with respect to valvular function at baseline. The design, with its unbiased treatment allocation, provides considerable evidence that dexfenfluramine was a causal agent in the production of the valvulopathy that was seen in the dexfenfluramine-treated patients. As it was expected to, randomization successfully balanced the groups with regard to age, gender, race and body mass index at baseline. There is no reason to believe that baseline valve function would not have been balanced as well. The separation of treatment from patient characteristics inherent in the design should have minimized any effects of pre-existing valve disease. This clinical trial, even with its mid-stream change in endpoint, provides compelling evidence about the role of dexfenfluramine over and above other potentially confounding factors as a cause of valvulopathy, because of the high inferential strength of the study design. If other risk factors for heart-valve disease had existed – even unknown ones as had been proposed to explain the findings in previous observational studies – it would not have mattered. The treatment was administered in a randomized fashion that had no relationship with any patient characteristics, known or unknown.

Randomized trials are considered to be the strongest research designs because of the complete independence of treatment effects from other effects that might influence the outcome. They are considered to be an experimental study design, because control over treatment allocation resides with the study protocol. Randomized trials are always prospective. They go forward in time from the assignment of a treatment to the development of an outcome – it is not possible to allocate a randomly assigned treatment at a time in the past.

Major disadvantages of randomized trials are that they are expensive, they take a long time to conduct, and they are carried out on highly selected population subsets. The high degree of selectivity may limit the ability of clinical trials to explain the effects of treatments once the treatments are released to more heterogeneous real-world clinic populations. Randomized trials require specially trained personnel, usually several of them, elaborate procedures for randomizing treatment, and may take months or years to conduct. Another limitation of the method is that randomized trials cannot be used to evaluate exposures (i.e., treatments) that are expected to be harmful. If we wanted to evaluate the risk of lifetime cigarette addiction based on age at which high-school students started smoking, the strongest scientific method would be to randomize high-school students of different ages to cigarette smoking. Ethical issues would outweigh scientific ones in this sort of circumstance, however, and (hopefully) no study that randomizes participants to treatments that are known to be harmful will ever be done.

The next strongest study design is that of the cohort study, which, like the clinical trial, uses a prospective design. The major difference between cohort studies and clinical trials is that cohort studies are observational studies, as opposed to clinical experiments. Observational studies investigate treatments or exposures as they occur naturally in populations, rather than allocate the treatments on the basis of an experimental design. Selection to a medical treatment for cohort studies is based on combinations of patient preferences, physician judgment, insurance coverage, and other social and cultural phenomena. For exposure studies of things other than medical treatment, populations usually self-select into risk groups by circumstances or lifestyle choices. Some teenagers smoke, some do not, some people work around hazardous chemicals, some do not, some people get regular exercise, some people do not, and so on. Many treatments or exposures – particularly those related to lifestyle factors – are very difficult to control in terms of allocating them to patients. Randomization (or any other experimental technique for that matter) cannot practically allocate such treatments or exposures. Cohort studies are next-best prospective studies that are most appropriately used when randomized treatment allocation is impractical or unethical. Cohort studies identify a treatment or exposure prior to the onset of an outcome in a population of patients who are free of the outcome at the time they are enrolled in the study. The main statistic in a cohort study is incidence, or the rate at which new cases of an outcome arise in the study sample during the study period. Measures of association between the outcome rate and the risk factors can be computed in cohort studies, and this makes cohort data quite valuable for use in risk studies. Although they do not have the benefit of randomization, ideally the treatment or exposure groups in a cohort study will be roughly comparable, and good information on important risk factors will be available for all groups. Risk factor information needs to be available so that statistical adjustments for the multiple risk factors can be made. In traditional cohort studies, the confounding effects of variables are controlled using mathematical models in order to focus and separate the effects of the main risk factor variable of interest from the effects of the other risk factors. In general, risk factors are not independent of one another with respect to outcome, so they all need to be considered together in order to determine how they co-operate to influence the probability that the outcome of interest will occur. Although the cohort design is prospective in terms of its "directionality" – in the sense that it ascertains exposure prior to outcome and looks forward in time to outcome – cohort studies can be assembled retrospectively if reliable data are available. Most studies of coronary bypass mortality, for example, are actually conducted after the outcomes under study have occurred. Hospital charts provide fairly reliable information on the risk factors that were present prior to surgery, and the outcome is well defined and clearly determinable postoperatively. Patients only undergo heart surgery if they are alive, so it is a good bet that mortality is either intraoperative or postoperative. Therefore, even though the risk factor and event may have occurred prior to assembly of the data for the study cohort, it is possible to construct a study that has prospective directionality from events that have already occurred. Studies of this type are known as *historical* cohort studies.

The major weaknesses of cohort studies are lack of randomization and inefficiency for rare events. Lack of randomization is a weakness because treatment or exposure may be tied to other factors. Smoking may be related to socioeconomic status, which may in turn be related to cancer mortality. Fortunately, good mathematical techniques and high-capacity computers can assist in the separation of such tangled effects, *as long as the presence and magnitude of the additional risk factors are measured and modeled accurately*. Unfortunately, it is never really possible to measure all additional risk factors that could be contributing to outcome. Therefore, efforts to identify and measure particularly strong influential variables should be made. Control for confounding requires that influential variables have actually been measured, since the effects of variables not measured cannot be estimated. Prospective designs, including both cohort studies and clinical trials, are inefficient for studying risk associated with rare outcomes. Prospective studies of risk factors for childhood leukemia, for example, whether randomized or not, would require the enrollment and follow-up of hundreds of thousands of children to capture a few cases. Such studies would be extremely expensive and would contribute very little information given their cost because of the low statistical power that would result from the small number of cases. For rare outcomes, case–control designs are usually preferred.

Case–control studies occupy the third tier in the hierarchy of study design strength (Table 3.2). Case–control studies involve the identifi-

**Table 3.2** Study designs: strengths and weaknesses

| Design | Strengths | Weaknesses |
|---|---|---|
| Randomized trial | Experimental control of treatment separates treatment from patient characteristics. | Expensive.<br>Time consuming.<br>Rigid entry criteria may limit generalizability. |
| Cohort study | Prospective design minimizes bias.<br>Can be used to study harmful exposures and real-life "usual care" situations. | Not randomized.<br>Time consuming. |
| Case–control | Increased efficiency for discovering risk factors, especially in rare event situations. | Prevalence-based: not directly interpretable in terms of risk.<br>Susceptible to many types of bias. |

cation of roughly equal groups of cases (people who have experienced a particular outcome, say, childhood leukemia) and a roughly comparable group of people who have not. If we wanted to know whether electromagnetic fields generated by high-tension power lines near the home were associated with elevated childhood leukemia risk, for example, we would assemble a group of children with leukemia and a group of children without, and measure the proximity of their homes to power lines. This approach would be much more efficient numerically, because approximately half the study sample would be children who actually had the disease. In order to identify them as cases, the children with leukemia would have to already have the diagnosis, and therefore they would be prevalent, as opposed to incident, cases. Prevalence is the proportion of a population that has a disease or outcome at a given time, while incidence is the rate at which new cases arise. Case–control studies are prevalence studies, which start with prevalent disease and look backward in time to risk factors that may be associated with the disease.

Case–control studies are generally more subject to bias than the prospective designs. Because the disease is prevalent at the time the study is conducted, past exposures that may be important are usually somewhat remote in time. This, in combination with recall bias, may seriously affect the validity of case–control results. Parents of children with leukemia may rack their brains trying to remember any little detail that might help to explain their child's unfortunate circumstances, and their memory of their child's remote exposure history may be different from that of parents whose children do not have leukemia. This can lead to differential reporting of potential exposures between groups and can cause risk factor prevalences between the groups to be reported inaccurately. Because of problems associated with measuring risk factors for prevalent conditions, occasionally case–control studies are done using incident case data. For relatively common conditions, it may be possible for investigators to use case–control methods to study newly diagnosed (incident) cases of disease. These are usually done in the context of ongoing cohort studies, and have the primary advantage of reducing the number of measurements that need to be done on the non-cases. Such studies are known as nested case–control studies.

Both types of case–control studies rely on the accrual of participants based on their case or non-case status rather than on their exposure profile. Even case–control studies that are nested in cohort studies do this, and as a result they change the proportion of cases relative to non-cases that occur in the cohort. Since risk in the risk-stratification situation is defined as long-term relative frequency, and relative frequency is defined as the frequency of events relative to the frequency of chances for an event to occur, the case–control design cannot be used to calculate risk directly. That is, risk is the ratio of events to the total number of chances that an event occurs. Chances and events lose their original relationship in case–control studies because of the way cases are accrued. Logistic regression analysis is used commonly in case–control studies as a method of control for confounding. But the results of a case–control study logistic regression analysis converted to probability would not reflect the type of population risk we would be after in a risk study. Case–control designs deal with disease as a prevalent condition, and are not appropriate for estimating risk. Case–control studies can be very useful for identifying risk *factors*, however, because they artificially increase the proportion of events that occur in the study population and therefore increase statistical power to a level that would take orders of magnitude more patients in prospective studies to match. Case–control findings, at least where risk studies are concerned, are best used to generate hypotheses about risk factors that can be confirmed in prospective studies.

Cross-sectional studies are the last design we will consider here. These are "quick and dirty" hypothesis-generating studies that examine the association between risk factors and outcomes at a single point, or cross-section, in time. The advantage of these studies is that they can be done quickly and can help to rough out hypotheses regarding the relationship between risk factors and outcomes. Their major limitation is that, because they are done at a single time point, it may not be possible to determine whether a risk factor existed prior to the onset of an outcome or whether it occurred afterwards. Cross-sectional studies are more reliable for mortality than other endpoints, because all risk factors would need to have occurred prior to death. But the reliability of cross-sectional studies decreases as the period of time between the exposure and the outcome increases. The longer someone can have had a disease or outcome, the more likely it is that supposed risk factors arose some time after the disease onset. Cross-sectional studies are of no value for risk analysis studies. In the hierarchy of evidence, only case reports and expert opinion fall below cross-sectional studies.

## Risk studies

Risk studies, because their aim is to make predictions about the future, are of necessity prospective, at least in "directionality". A prospective directionality, as we mentioned previously, means that the study looks from the presence of prior risk factors to the occurrence of an outcome. To arrive at risk, the outcome for *each and every* treated or exposed individual in a study population must be evaluated, because risk is defined as long-term relative frequency. Relative frequency, as we saw in Chapter 1, is the frequency of events relative to non-events. For this reason, it is a problem if events *or* non-events are missed. Missing data either way changes the relative frequencies of the estimates. Case–control studies, in contrast to prospective incidence studies, deliberately change the ratio of outcome to non-outcome groups in order to intensify the sensitivity of the mathematics to the effects of risk factors. As for risk study timing (as distinct from directionality), the actual measurements of risk factors and the outcome can be made before or after the outcome occurs in risk studies, in the same way that cohort studies can be prospective or historical.

Studies that are conducted with the intent that they function as risk-stratification studies are always prospective in directionality, although they may be historical in the timing of data collection. They are ordinarily cohort-type studies, with the major distinction that they do not focus on any risk factor in particular as the one of interest. A traditional cohort study of coronary bypass mortality, for example, might divide participants into two groups; say, those with chronic obstructive pulmonary disease (COPD) and those without, to determine whether COPD increases the risk of mortality following surgery. In order to determine this, it would be necessary, in addition to measuring the effects of COPD, to measure the effects of other things that might be related to both COPD and mortality following bypass surgery. Such common factors might include the extent of coronary stenosis, congestive heart failure, and other factors that are related to mortality and also to COPD via cigarette smoking. Multivariate analysis would permit the mathematical separation of the effect of COPD from the other confounding effects, so that the *independent* contribution of COPD to mortality following bypass surgery could be estimated. A risk-stratification study, on the other hand, though it might use exactly the same statistical analysis with exactly the same variables, would not attach any particular priority to the independent effects of COPD. The primary goal of risk stratification is prediction, rather than identification and isolation of the unique contributions of any particular variable. Multivariate analysis for risk stratification is designed to maximize the accuracy of the predictions by adjusting for non-independence between the predictors, rather than to make adjustments for use in the interpretation of predictor variable estimates.

> **→ TIP 3**
>
> Risk-stratification studies, unlike traditional clinical research studies, do not focus on the effect of a single predictive factor.

> **→ TIP 4**
>
> The goal of multivariate risk stratification is to maximize predictive accuracy rather than to adjust for confounding.

Although it would be possible to use exactly the same analysis for a traditional primary risk factor cohort study and a multivariate risk-stratification study, as a practical matter, this would be uncommon. Cohort studies are usually concerned as much with rate as with risk, and as a consequence they use statistical methods that take time into account as well as event probability. Statistical methods for time-to-event analyses are known as failure-time statistics, and commonly include the Kaplan–Meier method for univariate stratified analysis, and the Cox or proportional-hazards regression method for multivariable estimates. The Kaplan–Meier method is a method of calculating cumulative incidence – the rate that events arise over time – with allowance for a type of incompleteness known as censoring. In a five-year study of patient well-being after radiation therapy for cancer, for example, we might want to know what the incidence of local recurrence is. The most obvious way to do that would be to count up the recurrences over five years and compare that to the non-recurrences – that is, compute the five-year relative frequency or rate. But in practice it is not usually possible to make this simple calculation. For example, it is common for people who have had cancer to die from distant metastasis without the cancer recurring in the original site. Or it may be that some patients have only been on-study for three years and would not have a five-year follow-up. Kaplan–Meier allows us to use all the information contributed by these incomplete patient observations by keeping them in the at-risk but not-recurred group for as long as we know their status. When patients die, are lost to follow-up or run out of follow-up time, we remove them from the at-risk group at that time. This is the process known as censoring. Cox regression, also called proportional-hazards regression, is a multivariate extension of Kaplan–Meier that allows for multivariate testing of risk factors over cumulative incidence distributions that have censored data.

Risk studies, although they are a form of cohort study, are more likely to use logistic regression analyses, which model only the probability *that* an event will occur over a given time period – but not the *rate* at which the event occurs within that time period. This is a subtle distinction from Kaplan–Meier and Cox techniques, but it has major implications for transformation of a risk factor profile into the probability that an event will occur. Although the reasons for this are complex, a simple explanation is sufficient for our purposes here. It is difficult and not very reliable to use a risk factor profile to predict both the *probability* that an event will occur and the *time* that it will occur. It makes more sense for mathematical reasons to predict the probability that an event will occur within a certain time *period* than that it will occur at a particular time. Where traditional cohort studies ultimately want to estimate the difference in the rate of outcome occurrence based on a primary adjusted risk factor, risk-stratification studies want to use a constellation of risk factors to back-calculate risk for other populations. Logistic regression analysis, though it is used in risk-stratification studies for back-calculating risk expectations from risk factors, is also used widely in case–control studies in epidemiology, because it is well-suited to making adjusted inferences about the prevalence of risk factors in diseased and non-diseased groups. For this reason, many people associate logistic regression with case–control studies. But when probability can be handled as probability over a time period, logistic regression, with the probability transformation we described in Chapter 1, is a very effective way to compute multivariate risk. In Chapter 4 we will go through this process in detail, and will work examples that show each step in the process of calculating local risk from published standard logistic equations.

## Determining the appropriateness of a reference population

As we have seen, with regard to study design, numerous approaches can be taken to examine questions of the association between risk factor and outcome. Not all study designs are equal, however, when it comes to the directness of inferences that are derived from the predictor variables. Clinical trials and cohort studies are concerned with incidence – the rate at which an outcome arises in a population with a certain risk factor or constellation of risk factors. These are generally directly translatable to risk-stratification studies. Case–control studies, on the other hand, are concerned with prevalence, and with maximizing statistical power by making rare outcomes disproportionately more prevalent to non-case outcomes than they would be in nature if followed prospectively. Case–control studies, even those that are nested in cohort studies, do not provide data on incidence. For this reason, case–control studies are not directly interpretable as risk-stratification studies. The presence of a logistic regression analysis in a published study does not guarantee that the logistic equation will be useful for computing risk. The design and directionality of the study are major factors in determining the appropriateness of a study for use in risk stratification.

Ordinarily, the safest way to obtain appropriate risk-estimating equations is to get them from dedicated risk-stratification studies. Studies intended to produce such estimates and to produce interpretable observed/expected ratios are available in many areas of medicine, and some are even considered to be landmarks in particular areas. The New York State model for estimating mortality following bypass surgery is one such example. Landmark studies are not only usually high-quality studies – they serve as a standard by which other similar studies are judged. Estimates from landmark work may need to be included in reports on the topic that they cover, even when the research question is somewhat different and other risk equations that are deemed more appropriate are being applied as well. Many other considerations beyond study design influence the decision investigators must make when evaluating studies for use as risk-stratification standards.

Similarity of the research question between the published risk-stratification study and the local one being planned should be the first criterion for selection of a standard. The expectations that will ultimately be produced by the standard will only be meaningful if the local data question is the same. If the local question is "what is our center's expected *hospital* coronary bypass mortality risk?", it would be odd to select a study of *intra-operative* mortality as a standard. A published report of risk factors for intra-operative death would underestimate the hospital mortality experience of a local population, because most deaths following bypass surgery during the period of hospitalization do not occur in the operating room. Related to the research question are the case/non-case definition and the definitions of the predictor variables. In the intra-operative mortality example, all deaths in the operating room are cases. In the hospital mortality example, all deaths before hospital discharge are cases. So even though death is a common endpoint, the definition of what constitutes a case is different in these two examples. Because it affects all study inferences, the definition of what is and is not a case must be established in the standard study, and the same definition must be used in the local study. We covered case definition and case ascertainment in detail in Chapter 2, but it bears repeating here that the appropriateness of the study used as a standard for local risk adjustment is heavily dependent on the case definition.

Another important consideration in study selection is the similarity of the underlying population characteristics in the local population to the characteristics of the population being used as a standard. Some leeway in the prevalence of risk factors between the populations is natural – if it weren't, the population risk factor distributions would be identical and risk stratification would not be necessary. But major differences between the group upon which the standard equation is based and the local group being brought into conformance with the standard can be a problem, particularly when such differences are not measured. We said previously that control for confounding in clinical efficacy studies is only possible when the potentially confounding variables have been measured or when randomization has been employed. The same is true for risk-stratification studies. While risk stratification does not concern itself much with priority among measured variables, which is how confounding is usually described in conventional clinical research, risk estimates can be dramatically affected by unmeasured risk factors. We might think of these unmeasured variables as the confounders of risk stratification. As we will see in the next chapter, when the effects of a risk factor have been taken into account by risk stratification, any differences that remain between observed and expected events cannot be explained by the action of that particular risk factor. The effect of that risk factor has been adjusted out. But we have also said that any events that occur in a local population above what would be expected from a risk model are unexplained events. Because risk stratification is typically used to make inferences about quality of care, events that are not explained by risk models may be attributed to poor quality care. It is important, therefore, to understand what other differences might remain between a local population and a standard one after the risk factors in the risk model have been accounted for that could be responsible for remaining unexplained variation.

> **→ TIP 5**
>
> Risk-stratification studies usually assume that variation in outcome beyond what is predicted from risk factors is due to quality of care. For this reason, attention to other sources of unexplained variation when modeling risk is essential.

Our group consulted with an institution a few years ago in the area of hospital mortality risk following coronary bypass surgery using the New York State equation. At one point, expected risk was considerably lower than that observed in the population we were evaluating, even though all of the New York model variables had been accounted for. Further investigation into the matter showed that a large number of combined coronary bypass/carotid endarterectomy operations had been done in the local population we were looking at, and that these operations represented about eight percent of the total operations done in the time period of interest. We called the New York State Department of Health and they told us that they do not exclude such concomitant operations from their population, but that the prevalence of such operations in their population was less than one percent. As it turned out, the indication for combined operation at the institution we were working with was severe coronary artery and carotid disease, which the surgeons felt would be unsafe to handle in a staged operation. When we excluded the combined operations from the population, the actual results fell back into line with the results that were expected by the New York model. So the unmeasured effect of combined coronary bypass/carotid endarterectomy surgery explained all the excess mortality at that institution. The combination of the very different prevalences (eight percent versus less than one percent), the probable differences in indications for surgery (New York would probably either have measured or excluded these cases if the severe-disease indication were used there), and the fact that the risk factor was not measured all made the New York model inappropriate for predicting risk in the local population when the coronary bypass/carotid endarterectomies were left in.

Population characteristics are critical considerations in determining the appropriateness of a risk equation for producing expectations about a local population. If the populations are very different, the expectations will not reflect the legitimate experience of the local group. Since disparities between predicted results and actual ones are often viewed as reflecting institutional quality of care, the population chosen as a yardstick will affect the conclusions that are ultimately drawn from the data.

## Studies that can be used for risk measurements

Whenever it is possible, dedicated risk studies should be used for risk-stratification work. Occasionally, formal risk-stratification studies will

4

# Applying published risk estimates to local data

In this chapter, we discuss the application of published risk estimates to local data. Physicians have known for many years that crude comparisons of treatment outcomes between populations of patients are difficult to interpret because of the heterogeneity among populations with respect to underlying patient risk. Risk-stratification techniques were developed to help account for differences between populations that are attributable to risk factors, in order to facilitate meaningful comparison of the populations. Because of the increasing popularity of risk adjustment in the contemporary health-care environment, risk estimates are available from the literature for many different clinical problems. Published risk studies provide an external reference standard to which local results can be compared. The comparisons that are made between populations in risk-stratification studies are risk-adjusted comparisons that explain part of the variation in outcome between populations as a function of the risk factors that are present in the populations. Risk-adjusted comparisons provide for a more realistic comparison of population outcome than crude comparisons alone.

## Standardization of rates

All risk stratification involves the mathematical standardization of rates. A rate is simply the accumulation of new events over time. Cancer death rates per year, college student meningitis rates per semester, nursing home nosocomial infection rates per week – all of these rates are events over time, and all could be described by some sort of standardization or stratification procedure. The term "rate" is often applied informally to events that occur over a period without a fixed time interval, such as the period of hospitalization following coronary artery bypass surgery. Although the period of time spent in hospital after coronary bypass surgery may range from a few days to a month or more in extreme circumstances, so that there is not a fixed time interval over which events can occur, we can still think of events that occur during the hospitalization as rates in the sense that we would need to use them to perform rate standardization. It is occasionally troublesome to call proportions rates when they do not precisely describe incidence over a fixed unit of time, but this is mainly the case when *incidence* is confused with *prevalence.* Incidence describes all new cases of a problem that arise in a population over a defined period, while prevalence describes all the prevailing cases at a particular time point. This distinction is mostly a problem for diseases that people can have for a long period of time, because counting pre-existing cases among those that arise in a population over time can lead to incorrect estimates of incidence and to inappropriate conclusions about the effects of risk factors on disease onset rates. In cases where death is the study endpoint, the incidence/prevalence distinction is less of a problem, because people for whom death is a prevalent condition at the baseline are rarely enrolled in studies. Still, it is important to understand the distinction between incidence and prevalence and to pay attention to it when comparing groups. The conclusions drawn from incidence and prevalence studies – even of the same disease – can be quite different. For a more detailed discussion of issues regarding the validity of comparisons, see Chapter 3.

**Incidence**
The appearance of new cases of an event or outcome over a specified period of time. Also the rate at which new cases arise in a population.

**Prevalence**
A proportion that describes the relative frequency of a condition in a population at a particular point in time.

Rate standardization is essentially a process of gathering the results of a group or groups, taking the distribution of their characteristics into account, and bringing the groups against a common standard so that their outcomes can be compared. Stratum-specific rates are applied to a fixed factor, say the sample size for an age stratum for a given year, and a summary rate is computed from the estimates of the stratum rates adjusted for sample size. When several study samples are standardized to a particular variable, such as age, the effect of that variable on the overall outcome estimate is accounted for. This is very important, because it is the rationale for undertaking any standardization or stratification procedure. Any difference between two or more populations that exists following standardization *cannot be attributed to the standardization variable.* Standardization "adjusts out" the effect of a potentially confounding variable and allows for comparisons between groups to be made independently of the effect of the stratification variable. Age standardization to look at mortality across groups is a classic example. Table 4.1 shows the process of direct age standardization, which will make the concepts clearer.

This is a complicated table, so we will take it a bit at a time. The columns in the table, from left to right, are age (stratified into five-year increments except for the last two categories), estimated number of cancer deaths per age group in the year 1940, U.S. population in 1940 by age group, and the cancer mortality rate per 100,000 population in 1940 by age group (known as the stratum-specific mortality), estimated number of cancer deaths in the year 1980, stratum-specific U.S. population in 1980, stratum-specific cancer mortality rate in 1980. The last column is the number of deaths per stratum that would have been expected in 1980 if the population (using the 1980 rate per 100,000) had not changed from 1940. At the bottom of the table, again from left to right, are the estimated total number of cancer deaths in 1940, the total population in 1940, and a repeat of the same for 1980 in the next two columns. The last column is the total number of cancer deaths that would have been expected in the 1980 population *if the population had not changed* since 1940.

If we look below the table at the computations for 1940, we see that cancer mortality was 120.1 per 100,000 population. This is as compared to a rate of 183.8 per 100,000 in 1980. If we had only this information, we might worry that cancer rates had increased 53 percent in the U.S. population in 40 years, and this would be some cause for alarm. But we also know that United States demographics changed quite a bit over the 40 years between 1940 and 1980, mainly in that life expectancy has gone up. In 1940, slightly less than seven percent of the population was over 60 years of age. By 1980, this number had more than doubled to 16 percent. Since we know that fatal cancer is mainly a disease of older people, we might suspect that the shift in the age of the population could explain some of the apparent increase in the average population cancer mortality rate seen in the 1980 crude (un-adjusted) statistic. By using the 1940 population as a standard, and multiplying the stratum-specific

**Table 4.1** Direct age standardization of cancer rates in 1940 and 1980 U.S. populations

| | 1940 | | | 1980 | | | |
|---|---|---|---|---|---|---|---|
| Age | Deaths* | Population | Rate per 100,000 | Deaths* | Population | Rate per 100,000 | From 1940 Pop'n* |
| Under 5 | 495 | 10,541,000 | 4.7 | 687 | 16,348,000 | 4.2 | 443 |
| 5–9 | 321 | 10,685,000 | 3.0 | 785 | 16,700,000 | 4.7 | 502 |
| 10–14 | 341 | 11,746,000 | 2.9 | 711 | 18,242,000 | 3.9 | 458 |
| 15–19 | 493 | 12,334,000 | 4.0 | 1143 | 21,168,000 | 5.4 | 666 |
| 20–24 | 788 | 11,588,000 | 6.8 | 1534 | 21,319,000 | 7.2 | 834 |
| 25–29 | 1,287 | 11,097,000 | 11.6 | 2050 | 19,521,000 | 10.5 | 1,165 |
| 30–34 | 2,407 | 10,242,000 | 23.5 | 3038 | 17,561,000 | 17.3 | 1,771 |
| 35–39 | 4,143 | 9,545,000 | 43.4 | 4678 | 13,965,000 | 33.5 | 3,197 |
| 40–44 | 7,057 | 8,788,000 | 80.3 | 7783 | 11,669,000 | 66.7 | 5,862 |
| 45–49 | 11,012 | 8,255,000 | 133.4 | 14,228 | 11,090,000 | 128.3 | 10,591 |
| 50–54 | 15,167 | 7,257,000 | 209.0 | 26,804 | 11,710,000 | 228.9 | 16,611 |
| 55–59 | 18,111 | 5,844,000 | 309.9 | 41,605 | 11,615,000 | 358.2 | 20,933 |
| 60–64 | 20,959 | 4,728,000 | 443.3 | 53,043 | 10,088,000 | 525.8 | 24,860 |
| 65–74 | 44,327 | 6,377,000 | 695.1 | 127,437 | 15,581,000 | 817.9 | 52,158 |
| 75+ | 31,280 | 2,643,000 | 1183.5 | 130,963 | 9,969,000 | 1313.7 | 34,721 |
| Total | 158,188 | 131,670,000 | | 416,489 | 226,546,000 | | 174,772 |

1940 rate = 158,188/131,670,000 = 0.001201. 0.001201 × 100,000 = 120.1 per 100,000.

1980 rate = 416,489/226,546,000 = 0.001838. 0.001838 × 100,000 = 183.8 per 100,000.

1980 rate adjusted for 1940 population = 174,772/131,670,000 = 0.001327. 0.001327 × 100,000 = 132.7 per 100,000.

*Adapted from Hennekens and Buring (1) with permission.*

* Numbers of deaths are estimated in this example by multiplying population rate per 100,000 for each stratum by the stratum population weight. This is done to simplify the arithmetic involved in explaining the adjustment procedure. In a real population study, we would know the number of deaths and the population size, and would compute the rate per 100,000 from these two quantities.

1980 mortality rates against the corresponding age-group sample sizes from 1940, we obtain an average mortality rate in the 1940-distribution-adjusted 1980 population of 132.7 deaths per 100,000 population. This is much closer to the 1940 rate of 120.1 per 100,000 than was the crude 1980 estimate of 183.8 per 100,000. The age-adjusted excess mortality in the 1980 population is around 10.5 percent – about what we would expect to be due to increased smoking in the population between 1940 and 1980 (1).

The calculations go like this. In the first row of the third and fourth columns, we see that the 1940 population for the under 5 age group is 10,541,000. The cancer death rate is 4.7 per 100,000. To get the number of cases, we divide 4.7 (the incidence) by 100,000 (since incidence is expressed as per 100,000) to get 0.000047. We multiply the stratum sample size by this number to estimate the number of deaths. $0.000047 \times 10{,}541{,}000 = 495.4$. That number, rounded to 495, appears in column 2. We repeat the process for each stratum, and then sum the column of estimated deaths. This sums to 158,188 as shown at the bottom of the table. This number is divided by the total sample size for the 1940 population, which is 131,670,000. $158{,}188/131{,}670{,}000 = 0.001201$. Multiplied up by 100,000 we get 120.1 cases per 100,000 population, as shown below the table. The process works the same way for the 1980 group. To standardize the 1980 group to the 1940 group, the 1980 rates are multiplied against the 1940 sample sizes, the total taken, and an overall age-adjusted incidence of 132.7 per 100,000 is obtained.

In most real-life situations, the sample sizes and actual number of deaths are known, and it is necessary to compute the incidence rates per 100,000 by dividing the cases by the sample size. We show the process in reverse for all the data to minimize the amount of arithmetic, but multiplying rates from one group by sample sizes from another to get expected deaths is how the actual adjustment part of the process works.

## Multivariable risk stratification

Sometimes it is necessary to look at complex combinations of risk factors rather than only at one as with age above. While stratification techniques such as direct standardization are useful up to a point, when risk factors are multiple the number of strata becomes very large very quickly. This causes problems not only with the conceptualization and layout of the tables, but also leads to many risk factor strata with small samples, which makes the arithmetic troublesome as well. Multivariable regression techniques such as logistic regression analysis are powerful tools for making comparisons that involve complex risk factor problems. These techniques are able to generalize across groups of risk factors without the need for laying out all the possible combinations in tables.

As we saw in Chapter 1, logistic regression analysis uses a linear combination of risk factor values to estimate the dependence of a particular outcome on the risk factors. The estimate of the outcome likelihood is the logit, or the log odds. Statistically significant risk factor variables predict the odds of the outcome by accounting for more of the variance in outcome than can be explained by background variation alone. We will now go through an example of how a published logistic regression equation can be applied to local data to get an expected risk estimate.

As we saw in Chapter 1, the logistic regression model is of the form

$$o = \exp(\alpha + \beta_1 \chi_1 + \beta_2 \chi_2 \ldots \beta_n \chi_n)$$

where $o$ = odds, $\alpha$ is the model intercept term, $\beta_1$–$\beta_n$ are the model regression coefficients for risk factor variables 1–$n$, and $\chi_1$–$\chi_n$ are variable values that correspond to the model coefficients. Table 4.2, reproduced from Hannan *et al.* (2) with permission, lists variables and their logistic regression coefficients. This model was developed by the New York State Department of Health, and has been widely used to assess hospital mortality risk following coronary bypass surgery. To get an estimate of the risk we would expect for a patient based on the New York State model, we would multiply the patient's risk factor values through the model coefficients, sum the products, add the intercept and take the exponent. Table 4.3 shows the computational form of the equation, along with an example with patient data.

In this example we have a 72-year-old patient with no other risk factors. Note that all the non-age-related variables are "indicator" variables – with a value of 1 when they are present and zero when they are absent. Since multiplying regression coefficients by zero turns the value of the entire multiplied term to zero, as in our case of the 72-year-old

**Table 4.2** Predictor variables and logistic regression coefficients from the New York State model for prediction of coronary bypass hospital mortality

| Patient risk factors | Regression coefficient* | $p$ | OR (95% CI)† |
|---|---|---|---|
| Demographic | | | |
| Age, y‡ | 0.0346 | <0.0001 | 1.04 (1.03–1.04) |
| Age ≥70 y | 0.0439 | 0.0001 | 1.05 (1.03–1.07) |
| Female gender | 0.4154 | <0.0001 | 1.52 (1.36–1.69) |
| Coronary disease, left main stenosis >90% | 0.3612 | <0.0001 | 1.43 (1.23–1.67) |
| Reversible ischemia, unstable angina | 0.3533 | <0.0001 | 1.42 (1.27–1.60) |
| Left ventricular function | | | |
| Ejection fraction <0.20§ | 1.4008 | <0.0001 | 4.06 (3.16–5.21) |
| Ejection fraction 0.20–0.29§ | 0.7920 | <0.0001 | 2.21 (1.89–2.58) |
| Ejection fraction 0.30–0.39§ | 0.4881 | <0.0001 | 1.63 (1.43–1.86) |
| Ejection fraction missing | 0.4810 | <0.0001 | 1.62 (1.36–1.92) |
| Previous myocardial infarction within 7 d | 0.5253 | <0.0001 | 1.69 (1.45–1.97) |
| Preoperative intra-aortic balloon pump | 0.3284 | 0.0007 | 1.39 (1.15–1.68) |
| Congestive heart failure | 0.5684 | <0.0001 | 1.77 (1.53–2.04) |
| "Disasters" | 1.3814 | <0.0001 | 3.98 (3.12–5.08) |
| Comorbidities | | | |
| Diabetes | 0.4029 | <0.0001 | 1.50 (1.34–1.67) |
| Morbid obesity | 0.3961 | 0.0003 | 1.49 (1.20–1.84) |
| Chronic obstructive pulmonary disease | 0.3063 | <0.0001 | 1.36 (1.20–1.54) |
| Dialysis dependence | 1.0281 | <0.0001 | 2.80 (2.26–3.46) |
| Other, previous open heart operation | 1.3174 | <0.0001 | 3.73 (3.29–4.24) |

* Constant = −6.9605.

† OR indicates odds ratio; and CI, confidence interval.

‡ For age, the odds of a patient younger than 70 years dying in the hospital compared with the odds of a patient $n$ years younger dying in the hospital are $e^{n(0.0346)}$ times higher (e.g., the odds of a 65-year-old dying in the hospital are $e^{0.346} = 1.41$ times higher than the odds of a 55-year-old patient dying in the hospital, all other risk factors being the same). The odds of a patient older than 70 years dying in the hospital are $e^{n(0.0439)}$ times higher than a patient $n$ years younger but also older than 70 years. The odds of a patient of age $m$ (>70 years) dying in the hospital are $e^{(m-70)(0.0439)+n(0.0346)}$ times higher than the odds for a patient $n$ years younger but younger than 70 years. For example, the odds of a 75-year-old dying in the hospital are $e^{5(0.0439)+10(0.0346)} = 1.76$ times the odds of a 65-year-old dying in the hospital.

**Table 4.2 (*cont.*)**

§ For ejection fraction, the ORs for the three categories given are all relative to patients with ejection fractions ≥.40, the omitted category.
Adapted from Hannan *et al.* (1994) Improving the outcomes of coronary artery bypass surgery in New York State. *JAMA* **271**: 761–6, copyright 1994, American Medical Association.

**Table 4.3** The computational form of the New York State model

odds = exp[−6.9605 + (age × 0.0346) + (m70 × 0.0439) + (female × 0.4154) + (lmain × 0.3612) + (uangina × 0.3533) + (eflt20 × 1.4008) + (ef2029 × 0.7920) + (ef3039 × 0.4881) + (efmiss × 0.4810) + (recentmi × 0.5253) + (balpump × 0.3284) + (chf × 0.5684) + (disast × 1.3814) + (diabetes × 0.4029) + (mobesity × 0.3961) + (copd × 0.3063) + (dialysis × 1.0281) + (prevop × 1.3174)]

odds = exp[−6.9605 + (72 × 0.0346) + (2 × 0.0439)] = 0.01251
probability = 0.01251/1.01251 = 0.01235
percent = 0.01235 × 100 = 1.235

*Odds*, predicted odds of hospital mortality; −6.9605, the intercept term or constant; *age*, age in years; *m70*, number of years beyond age 70. All the other variables are indicator variables with a value of one if they are true (present) and zero if they are false (absent). *Female*, female gender; *lmain*, left main coronary artery stenosis greater than 90%; *uangina*, unstable angina; *eflt20*, left ventricular ejection fraction (LVEF) less than 20%; *ef2029*, LVEF between 20 and 29%; *ef3039*, LVEF between 30 and 39%; *efmiss*, missing value of LVEF; *recentmi*, myocardial infarction within seven days preoperatively; *balpump*, intra-aortic balloon pump *preoperatively*; *chf*, congestive heart failure; *disast*, the New York Department of Health's definition – a myocardial structural defect, acute renal failure or shock; *diabetes*, diabetes; *mobesity*, morbid obesity; *copd*, chronic obstructive pulmonary disease; *dialysis*, dialysis dependence; *prevop*, any history of a previous open heart operation.

In the example shown in the table, the patient is a 72-year-old male with no other risk factors. The value of the age variable is 72, the value of M70 is 2, and all the other indicator variable values are zero. The equation's solution for this patient simplifies to the intercept and the terms for age and M70.

man with no other risk factors, the model simplifies to the intercept, the term for age and the term for years beyond 70. The rest of the equation amounts to adding up 16 zeroes, so we can just drop any terms that have zero indicator variable values. To get odds in this example, we multiply age and years of age beyond 70 by their respective regression coefficients, add these two products together, add the negative intercept (subtracting it would be equivalent mathematically, but we show this form of the equation because it can be used with any logistic model regardless of the sign of the intercept), and take the exponent of the sum of the whole thing. In this case, odds work out to be 0.01251, or, based on our discussion in Chapter 1, 80: 1 in favor of survival. Probability, as we recall from Chapter 1, is computed from odds as $p = o/(1 + o)$ (equation 1.1), so in this case probability = 0.01251/1.01251 = 0.01235. Raised to percent the expected probability of hospital mortality for this patient would be 1.235 percent based on the New York model.

**→ TIP 1**

Computers can solve many equations rapidly and without the errors common to hand calculations. Use a computer to solve equations whenever possible.

While logistic equations can readily be solved using a hand calculator, it is a great deal of trouble to do very many calculations that way. Fortunately, we have computer programs that can do calculations the same way for many patients, and this is by far the preferable way to do this sort of thing when more than a few cases are involved. For one, it's easier. For two, the likelihood of computational errors is vastly reduced, because once the program code is written and checked, the computer will do the calculations exactly the same way for each data record. Table 4.4 shows the SAS code that produced the example shown in Table 4.5. See Appendix 1 for a line-by-line explanation of the program.

## Calculation of expected risk for a study sample

Performing these computations on groups of patients allows for risk-adjusted comparisons to be made between groups, or for a single group to be compared against a standard. Ultimately, most risk-stratification projects are oriented toward one or both of these goals. To show how the risk-stratification procedure works for a group of patients, we read three years' worth of the coronary bypass experience of one of our authors (M.J.R.) into the program shown in Table 4.4. Table 4.5 shows the first 42 consecutive cases from this run (readers can follow the discussion

**Table 4.4** SAS program for solving the New York State Model used at our institutions, and used to produce Table 4.5. The program is described line-by-line in Appendix 1

```
data ch4;
infile 'd:\bookstat\ch4dat.txt' missover lrecl=265;
informat doadmit datesurg datedis mmddyy8.;
format doadmit datesurg datedis mmddyy8.;
input counter 1-10 encounte 12-26 lname$ 28-62 fname$ 64-98 surgeon$ 100-134
 drg 136-141 doadmit age 152-154 height 156-161 weight 163-168 female 170
 smoke 172 packs 174-179 yrs 181-186 lmain 188 uangina 190 sangina 192
 ptcaemer 194 ivnitr 196 ivinotr 198 ef 200-205 novessel 207 venaneu 209
 mi7d 211 mi24h 213 mi3wk 215 migt3wk 217 balpump 219 chf 221 structur 223
 renfail 225 shock 227 htn 229 diabetes 231 copd 233 dialysis 235 CVD 237
 valvdis 239 prevsurg 241 datesurg datedis death 261 priority 263;
htm=(height*2.54)/100;
wtk=weight/2.2;
bmi=wtk/(htm**2);
if bmi ge 39 then mobesity=1;else mobesity=0;
pyears=packs*yrs;
if smoke=1 and packs=0 then pyears=.;
if ef=0 then ef=.;
if ef gt  0 and ef lt 20 then eflt20=1;else eflt20=0;
if ef ge 20 and ef lt 30 then ef2029=1;else ef2029=0;
if ef ge 30 and ef lt 40 then ef3039=1;else ef3039=0;
if ef=. then efmiss=1;else efmiss=0;
if mi7d=1 or mi24h=1 then recentmi=1;else recentmi=0;
if prevsurg gt 0 then prevop=1;else prevop=0;
if age gt 70 then m70=age-70;
if age le 70 then m70=0;
if structur=1 or renfail=1 or shock=1 then disast=1;else disast=0;
mortodds=exp(-6.9605+(age*0.0346)+(m70*0.0439)+(female*0.4154)+
 (lmain*0.3612)+(uangina*0.3533)+(eflt20*1.4008)+(ef2029*0.7920)+
 (ef3039*0.4881)+(efmiss*0.4810)+(recentmi*0.5253)+(balpump*0.3284)+
 (chf*0.5684)+(disast*1.3814)+(diabetes*0.4029)+(mobesity*0.3961)+
 (copd*0.3063)+(dialysis*1.0281)+(prevop*1.3174));
probmort=mortodds/(1+mortodds);
pctmort=probmort*100;
run;
proc print;var age m70 female lmain uangina eflt20 ef2029 ef3039 efmiss recentmi
 balpump chf disast diabetes mobesity copd dialysis prevop mortodds probmort pctmort;
run;
```

with a calculator for a report this short if desired). The sample represents only diagnosis-related group 106 and 107 clean coronary bypasses – no valves or other heart or peripheral vascular procedures are included. The model is only designed to represent risk expectations for clean coronary bypasses.

Patient identifiers and date of surgery have been removed for confidentiality reasons. Table 4.5 shows the 18 New York Model risk factor variable values for each patient (explanation of the variable names is

**Table 4.5** Printout of the New York Model solution, showing model predictor data for each patient, predicted mortality odds, predicted mortality probability, and mortality probability raised to percent. This table was produced using the SAS code in Table 4.4.

The SAS System 14:10 Tuesday, September 28, 1999

| OBS | AGE | M70 | FEMALE | LMAIN | UANGINA | EFLT20 | EF2029 | EF3039 | EFMISS | RECENTMI | BALPUMP | CHF | DISAST | DIABETES | MOBESITY | COPD | DIALYSIS | PREVOP | DEATH | MORTODDS | PROBMORT | PCTMORT |
|---|---|---|---|---|---|---|---|---|---|---|---|---|---|---|---|---|---|---|---|---|---|---|
| 1 | 72 | 2 | 0 | 0 | 0 | 0 | 0 | 0 | 0 | 0 | 0 | 0 | 0 | 0 | 0 | 0 | 0 | 0 | 2 | 0.01251 | 0.01235 | 1.2352 |
| 2 | 65 | 0 | 0 | 0 | 1 | 0 | 0 | 0 | 0 | 0 | 0 | 0 | 0 | 0 | 0 | 0 | 0 | 0 | 2 | 0.01280 | 0.01264 | 1.2640 |
| 3 | 62 | 0 | 0 | 0 | 1 | 0 | 0 | 0 | 0 | 0 | 0 | 0 | 0 | 0 | 0 | 0 | 0 | 0 | 2 | 0.01154 | 0.01141 | 1.1408 |
| 4 | 56 | 0 | 0 | 0 | 1 | 0 | 0 | 0 | 0 | 0 | 0 | 0 | 0 | 0 | 0 | 0 | 0 | 0 | 2 | 0.00938 | 0.00929 | 0.9289 |
| 5 | 72 | 2 | 1 | 0 | 1 | 0 | 0 | 0 | 0 | 1 | 0 | 0 | 0 | 0 | 0 | 0 | 0 | 0 | 2 | 0.04562 | 0.04363 | 4.3626 |
| 6 | 55 | 0 | 1 | 0 | 0 | 0 | 0 | 0 | 0 | 0 | 0 | 0 | 0 | 0 | 0 | 0 | 0 | 0 | 2 | 0.00964 | 0.00955 | 0.9545 |
| 7 | 55 | 0 | 0 | 0 | 1 | 0 | 0 | 0 | 0 | 0 | 0 | 0 | 0 | 0 | 0 | 0 | 0 | 0 | 2 | 0.00906 | 0.00898 | 0.8976 |
| 8 | 65 | 0 | 0 | 0 | 0 | 0 | 0 | 0 | 0 | 0 | 0 | 0 | 0 | 0 | 0 | 0 | 0 | 0 | 2 | 0.00899 | 0.00891 | 0.8911 |
| 9 | 69 | 0 | 1 | 0 | 0 | 0 | 0 | 0 | 0 | 0 | 0 | 1 | 0 | 1 | 0 | 0 | 0 | 0 | 2 | 0.04132 | 0.03968 | 3.9681 |
| 10 | 65 | 0 | 0 | 0 | 0 | 0 | 0 | 0 | 0 | 0 | 0 | 0 | 0 | 0 | 0 | 0 | 0 | 0 | 2 | 0.00899 | 0.00891 | 0.8911 |
| 11 | 66 | 0 | 0 | 0 | 0 | 0 | 0 | 0 | 0 | 0 | 0 | 0 | 0 | 1 | 0 | 0 | 0 | 0 | 2 | 0.01393 | 0.01373 | 1.3735 |
| 12 | 73 | 3 | 1 | 0 | 1 | 0 | 0 | 0 | 0 | 0 | 0 | 0 | 0 | 0 | 0 | 0 | 0 | 0 | 2 | 0.02918 | 0.02835 | 2.8352 |
| 13 | 54 | 0 | 0 | 0 | 1 | 0 | 0 | 0 | 1 | 0 | 0 | 0 | 0 | 1 | 0 | 0 | 0 | 0 | 2 | 0.02118 | 0.02074 | 2.0737 |
| 14 | 73 | 3 | 0 | 0 | 0 | 0 | 0 | 0 | 0 | 0 | 0 | 1 | 0 | 1 | 0 | 0 | 0 | 0 | 2 | 0.03573 | 0.03450 | 3.4500 |
| 15 | 67 | 0 | 0 | 0 | 1 | 1 | 0 | 0 | 0 | 0 | 0 | 0 | 0 | 0 | 0 | 0 | 0 | 1 | 2 | 0.20788 | 0.17210 | 17.2102 |
| 16 | 65 | 0 | 0 | 0 | 1 | 0 | 0 | 1 | 0 | 1 | 1 | 1 | 0 | 1 | 0 | 0 | 0 | 1 | 1 | 0.48302 | 0.32570 | 32.5700 |
| 17 | 74 | 4 | 0 | 0 | 1 | 0 | 0 | 0 | 1 | 0 | 0 | 0 | 0 | 0 | 0 | 1 | 0 | 1 | 2 | 0.17093 | 0.14598 | 14.5978 |
| 18 | 75 | 5 | 0 | 0 | 1 | 0 | 0 | 0 | 0 | 0 | 0 | 0 | 0 | 0 | 0 | 0 | 0 | 1 | 2 | 0.08414 | 0.07761 | 7.7608 |
| 19 | 76 | 6 | 1 | 0 | 1 | 0 | 0 | 0 | 0 | 0 | 0 | 0 | 1 | 0 | 0 | 0 | 0 | 0 | 1 | 0.14699 | 0.12815 | 12.8152 |
| 20 | 72 | 2 | 0 | 0 | 0 | 0 | 0 | 0 | 0 | 0 | 0 | 0 | 0 | 0 | 0 | 0 | 0 | 0 | 2 | 0.01251 | 0.01235 | 1.2352 |
| 21 | 89 | 19 | 1 | 1 | 1 | 0 | 0 | 0 | 0 | 1 | 0 | 0 | 0 | 1 | 0 | 0 | 0 | 0 | 2 | 0.37199 | 0.27113 | 27.1129 |
| 22 | 67 | 0 | 0 | 0 | 1 | 0 | 1 | 0 | 0 | 1 | 1 | 1 | 1 | 1 | 0 | 0 | 0 | 0 | 2 | 0.74781 | 0.42786 | 42.7857 |
| 23 | 67 | 0 | 0 | 0 | 0 | 0 | 0 | 0 | 0 | 0 | 0 | 0 | 0 | 1 | 0 | 0 | 0 | 0 | 2 | 0.01442 | 0.01421 | 1.4211 |
| 24 | 55 | 0 | 0 | 0 | 0 | 0 | 0 | 0 | 1 | 0 | 0 | 0 | 0 | 0 | 0 | 0 | 0 | 0 | 2 | 0.01029 | 0.01019 | 1.0186 |
| 25 | 79 | 9 | 0 | 0 | 0 | 0 | 1 | 0 | 0 | 0 | 0 | 1 | 0 | 0 | 0 | 0 | 0 | 0 | 2 | 0.08445 | 0.07787 | 7.7873 |
| 26 | 67 | 0 | 0 | 0 | 0 | 0 | 0 | 0 | 1 | 0 | 0 | 0 | 0 | 1 | 0 | 0 | 0 | 0 | 2 | 0.02332 | 0.02279 | 2.2790 |
| 27 | 74 | 4 | 1 | 0 | 1 | 0 | 0 | 0 | 0 | 0 | 0 | 0 | 0 | 1 | 0 | 0 | 0 | 0 | 2 | 0.04722 | 0.04509 | 4.5092 |
| 28 | 59 | 0 | 0 | 0 | 0 | 0 | 0 | 0 | 0 | 0 | 0 | 0 | 0 | 1 | 0 | 0 | 0 | 0 | 2 | 0.01093 | 0.01081 | 1.0812 |
| 29 | 55 | 0 | 0 | 0 | 1 | 0 | 0 | 0 | 0 | 0 | 0 | 0 | 0 | 1 | 0 | 0 | 0 | 1 | 2 | 0.05060 | 0.04816 | 4.8159 |
| 30 | 66 | 0 | 0 | 0 | 0 | 0 | 0 | 0 | 0 | 0 | 0 | 0 | 0 | 0 | 0 | 0 | 0 | 1 | 2 | 0.03475 | 0.03359 | 3.3585 |
| 31 | 68 | 0 | 0 | 0 | 1 | 0 | 0 | 0 | 1 | 0 | 0 | 0 | 0 | 0 | 0 | 0 | 0 | 0 | 2 | 0.02297 | 0.02246 | 2.2458 |
| 32 | 51 | 0 | 0 | 0 | 0 | 0 | 0 | 0 | 0 | 0 | 0 | 0 | 0 | 1 | 0 | 0 | 0 | 0 | 2 | 0.00829 | 0.00822 | 0.8219 |
| 33 | 61 | 0 | 0 | 0 | 1 | 0 | 0 | 0 | 0 | 0 | 0 | 0 | 0 | 0 | 0 | 0 | 0 | 0 | 2 | 0.01115 | 0.01102 | 1.1024 |
| 34 | 59 | 0 | 0 | 1 | 0 | 0 | 0 | 0 | 0 | 0 | 0 | 0 | 0 | 1 | 0 | 0 | 0 | 1 | 2 | 0.05857 | 0.05533 | 5.5326 |
| 35 | 51 | 0 | 0 | 0 | 0 | 0 | 0 | 0 | 0 | 0 | 0 | 0 | 0 | 1 | 0 | 0 | 0 | 0 | 2 | 0.00829 | 0.00822 | 0.8219 |
| 36 | 78 | 8 | 0 | 0 | 1 | 0 | 0 | 1 | 0 | 0 | 0 | 0 | 0 | 1 | 0 | 0 | 0 | 0 | 2 | 0.06952 | 0.06500 | 6.4998 |
| 37 | 79 | 9 | 0 | 0 | 0 | 0 | 0 | 0 | 0 | 0 | 0 | 0 | 0 | 0 | 0 | 0 | 0 | 0 | 2 | 0.02167 | 0.02121 | 2.1207 |
| 38 | 70 | 0 | 1 | 0 | 0 | 0 | 0 | 0 | 0 | 0 | 0 | 1 | 0 | 1 | 0 | 0 | 0 | 0 | 2 | 0.04278 | 0.04102 | 4.1020 |
| 39 | 62 | 0 | 0 | 0 | 0 | 0 | 0 | 1 | 0 | 0 | 0 | 0 | 0 | 0 | 0 | 0 | 0 | 0 | 2 | 0.01320 | 0.01303 | 1.3032 |
| 40 | 66 | 0 | 0 | 0 | 0 | 0 | 0 | 0 | 0 | 0 | 0 | 0 | 0 | 0 | 0 | 0 | 0 | 0 | 2 | 0.00931 | 0.00922 | 0.9222 |
| 41 | 79 | 9 | 0 | 0 | 0 | 0 | 0 | 0 | 0 | 0 | 0 | 0 | 0 | 0 | 0 | 0 | 0 | 0 | 2 | 0.02167 | 0.02121 | 2.1207 |
| 42 | 57 | 0 | 0 | 0 | 0 | 0 | 0 | 0 | 0 | 0 | 0 | 0 | 0 | 0 | 0 | 0 | 0 | 0 | 2 | 0.00682 | 0.00677 | 0.6771 |

found in the legend for Table 4.3), whether or not the patient died in hospital (1 = yes, 2 = no), the odds calculated from the logistic regression equation (mortodds), the predicted probability of mortality (probmort), and the probability as a percent (pctmort).

Multivariate risk adjustment in patient groups is similar to the age standardization we saw at the beginning of this chapter, in that it produces an aggregated expected risk based on the profile of risk factors in the study sample. To calculate risk that is predicted by the regression model, we simply calculate the average risk for the sample by adding up all the predicted risk values and dividing by the total number of patients. For example, if Table 4.5 were our sample population, we would add up the risk numbers in the column labeled "probmort", and divide the total by 42, which is the number of patients. The total of the "probmort" column is 2.37. Divided by 42, we get an average expected risk of 0.0564, or 5.64 percent. We can convert this average to expected number of deaths in the sample by multiplying the average risk by the sample size. In this example, it would be $0.0564 \times 42 = 2.37$. The expected number of deaths is actually just the sum of the probabilities, because adding them up, dividing them by the sample size and then multiplying the dividend by the sample size is the same mathematically as just adding them up.

This process is substantially identical to the process we used in doing the direct age standardization at the beginning of this chapter. Here, we calculate stratum-specific rate (risk) estimates, with patient instead of age group as the stratum. In this case the risk calculation came from a multivariate logistic summary based on the model developed by the New York State Department of Health, instead of from U.S. vital statistics tables. Because each patient has one risk estimate it is not necessary to weight the estimates by stratum sample size as we did above. Weighting of the risk factors themselves as they occur within individual patients is taken care of by the logistic model. We aggregate the risk by adding it up over all the observations and then divide it by the sample size to get the average for the sample. We can multiply the average risk back up by the sample size to get the expected number of cases.

Finally, we can look at the number of patients that actually died in our study sample, and compare that to the number of deaths predicted by the model. In this example, we see that two patients actually died while

2.37 deaths were predicted by the model. So, after taking risk factors into account, the mortality observed in our sample is lower than what was expected by the model.

## The observed/expected ratio

> **➔ TIP 2**
>
> The *O/E* ratio quantifies the magnitude of the difference between observed events and expected ones.

To determine whether the number of deaths that actually occurred in a population is different from the number that would have been expected based on the risk factor profile, the observed number is divided by the expected number. This is known as the observed/expected or *O/E* ratio. Based on data from Table 4.5, the *O/E* ratio would be 2/2.37 = 0.84. If the *O/E* ratio is greater than one, more deaths are observed than the New York State model would have expected based on the risk factor profile in the study sample. Conversely, if the *O/E* ratio is less than one, observed mortality is less than would have been expected. Whether the difference between observed and expected is important is traditionally determined by statistical significance testing. Because dead or alive is a discrete variable that has only two possible values, statistical significance is governed by the chi-square distribution, which is a probability distribution for discrete data.

Table 4.6 shows the SAS code for calculating the *O/E* ratio, the 95% confidence interval for the *O/E* ratio, and the chi-square *p* value for the test. A line-by-line explanation for the program can be found in Appendix 2. The *p* value tells us what the probability is that we would observe a difference between observed and expected outcomes that is as extreme or more extreme than the difference we actually observe. In our example of the data from Table 4.5, where two deaths are observed and 2.37 are expected, the *O/E* ratio is 0.84 as we have seen. The formula for calculating the chi-square distribution quantile for the O/E ratio is shown in equation 4.1:

**Equation 4.1**

$$\chi^2 = (\text{observed} - \text{expected})^2/\text{expected}$$

In our example of observed = 2 and expected = 2.37, we would get $(2-2.37)^2/2.37 = 0.058$ which is chi-square distributed with one degree of freedom. The result of this calculation – in this example 0.058 – is the chi-square quantile, *not the p value.* The *p* value is the probability

**Table 4.6** SAS code for calculating an observed/expected ratio with 95% confidence intervals and chi square p value. This program is described line-by-line in Appendix 2

```
data oe;
input o e;
oeratio=o/e;
lci=(o*((1-(1/(9*o))-((1.96/3)*(sqrt(1/o))))**3))/e;
uci=((o+1)*((1-(1/(9*(o+1)))+((1.96/3)*(sqrt(1/(o+1)))))**3))/e;
x2=((o-e)**2)/e;
p=1-probchi(x2,1);
cards;
2 2.37
;
run;
proc print;run;
```

associated with the chi-square quantile. Most basic statistics books have chi-square tables in the back, and most statistical software, and even some spreadsheet programs, will compute the probability for a chi-square quantile. The probability ($p$ value) associated with the chi-square quantile 0.058 with one degree of freedom is 0.81. Ordinarily, the $p$ value would need to be less than 0.05 for us to conclude that a statistically significant difference is present. Since 0.81 is much larger than 0.05, we would conclude that 2 and 2.37 are not statistically significantly different from one another in this sample of 42 patients.

In addition to determining the statistical significance of a result from the $p$ value, we might also like to know how much variability is associated with the estimate. Confidence intervals are helpful in determining how much variation is present in the estimate, and they also give us an idea of what the average range of other $O/E$ ratios might be in repeated sampling with a group of this size. Confidence intervals at the 95% level have the property of excluding the null value ($O/E$ ratio $=1$) when the chi-square test is significant at $p<0.05$. So a lower 95% confidence interval above one or an upper 95% confidence interval below one would indicate a statistically significant $O/E$ ratio. The lower confidence limit is calculated thus:

**Table 4.7** Printout produced by SAS code in Table 4.6. O = observed cases, E = model expected cases, OERATIO = O/E ratio, LCI = lower 95% confidence interval, UCI = upper 95% confidence interval, χ2 = chi square quantile, P = chi-square probability

The SAS System 14:10 Tuesday, September 28, 1999

| OBS | O | E | OERATIO | LCI | UCI | χ2 | P |
|---|---|---|---|---|---|---|---|
| 1 | 2 | 2.37 | 0.84388 | 0.094774 | 3.04683 | 0.057764 | 0.81007 |

**Equation 4.2**

$$\text{LCL} = \text{observed} \times [1 - (1/9 \times \text{observed}) - (1.96/3) \times \sqrt{(1/\text{observed})}]^3 / \text{expected}$$

The upper confidence limit is:

**Equation 4.3**

$$\text{UCL} = (\text{observed} + 1) \times [1 - (1/9 \times (\text{observed} + 1)) + (1.96/3) \times \sqrt{(1/\text{observed} + 1))}]^3 / \text{expected}$$

A worked example is shown in Table 4.7, which is the output from the SAS code in Table 4.6. The SAS code (Table 4.6) shows the computational requirements for placement of parentheses so that the equation steps are executed in the proper order. The confidence interval formulas are from Rothman and Boice (3).

Before we leave the topic of significance testing, it is important that we have a concept of the importance of statistical power. Statistical power is the likelihood that we will be able to detect a difference if one actually exists. In the chi-square case, power is determined by the size of the sample, the frequency (or more importantly the rarity) of events, the size of the difference between the observed and the expected, and the alpha error level, also known as the *p* value, which is the statistical significance criterion (usually five percent, expressed as $p<0.05$). Comparisons that do not show statistical significance between observed and expected values may be non-significant as a result of low statistical power. In this case, it may not be appropriate to interpret non-significant results as showing equivalence between observed and expected outcomes. When sample sizes are small and observed differences are large, statistical power problems are of legitimate concern. A detailed treatment of statistical power is beyond the scope of this book. Interested readers are referred to Rosner (4) or to the many other introductory statistics texts that cover this topic. In general, though, some simple guidelines for dealing with power problems apply. First, results that are statistically significant cannot be criticized on the grounds that *statistical power* is low. Power is the inverse of type-2 statistical error, which states that an error has been made when an effect exists that is missed by the probability estimate. A result that is statistically significant is not missed – it is detected. So low power cannot be an explanation for a statistically significant result. Second, differences between observed and expected of twofold or more (*O*/*E* ratio of 2.0 for higher than expected results, 0.5 for lower than expected) are generally considered large, and should be detectable. Failure to detect a twofold result as being statistically significant probably indicates a problem with statistical power. A third guideline is that, for comparisons of low-incidence treatment results against a standard, a relatively large sample should be accrued before significance testing and interpretation are attempted. In the case of coronary bypass, for example, where deaths are generally expected to range from one to five percent depending on the type of practice, one or two events can make a percentage point difference in the percent actual mortality for populations as small as a couple of hundred. In a population of 100 patients, each death represents a single percentage point. The smaller the population being studied, the more influence each death has on the estimates.

**Statistical power**
The probability that a difference or association that really exists will be detected by a statistical test.

## Interpretation issues

It is worth pointing out that predictions made by risk models of this type (or any type for that matter) cannot be made with perfect accuracy. All the patients who survived in the example shown in Table 4.5 had some degree of expected risk. By the same token, the two who died each had expected risks less than 100 percent. Because there is inherent variability in biological systems, and because every conceivable risk factor is not included in a prediction model, a certain amount of model error will always be present. The term "model error" does not mean that the model is incorrect, it means only that the estimates are associated with a certain amount of variation beyond the model's power to explain. This problem is not restricted only to logistic regression models, but is a factor in all prediction modeling. Whether the goal is to forecast the path of a hurricane, predict the winner in the next presidential campaign, or predict death following coronary bypass surgery, uncertainty is a fact of life in the business of mathematical prediction. As we pointed out in Chapter 1, humans are biological creatures, and as such whether we live or die is subject to a fair amount of uncertainty. Some outcomes simply cannot be predicted beforehand, no matter how good our data. Explaining a death after the fact and predicting it in advance are entirely different matters. Most models constructed with biological data explain at best 30–50 percent of the variance in outcome. See Chapter 1 for a more detailed discussion of model error and prediction accuracy.

**➔ TIP 3**

95% confidence intervals are an essential part of interpreting the *O*/*E* ratio. They should always be reported when an *O*/*E* ratio is reported.

Some predictive uncertainty is attributable to sample size, as we mentioned above in the discussion of statistical power for *O*/*E* ratios. Interpretation of the results of an *O*/*E* ratio calculation is very dependent on statistical power. Confidence intervals should always be calculated for *O*/*E* ratios, because they are essential to interpretation of the results. Extremely wide confidence intervals (say, with a lower tail less that 0.3 and an upper tail of 10 or more) indicate poor predictability due to high statistical variation. In general, local risk-stratification efforts should not report *p* values for *O*/*E* ratios on small numbers. An informal guideline that has been used for several years in the risk stratification of coronary bypass mortality, for example, is that local results should not be evaluated using statistics until the numbers are in the range of 200–250 cases. Beyond that, individual physicians with fewer than 20–30 cases for the covered time period should not be evaluated statistically. Confidence intervals for observations made on small samples are extremely important for understanding power effects on the estimates, and *O*/*E* ratios on small samples should never be reported without them.

For widely studied problems, such as coronary bypass surgery, some generally accepted risk equations may have been applied to many individual data sets around the country or the world, and may even serve as a standard by which center-by-center results are judged. In the literature on coronary artery bypass surgery, the New York State Health Department's risk equation is a landmark standard. When contemplating a study of local data, one should always consider using data from other studies, if they are highly regarded and relevant, as benchmarks. Departures of the local population from appropriate use of such models, such as differences in research question, or variable or case definition, should always be discussed in reports that do not use the concept area standard. Any coronary bypass mortality study that were to be published currently would be criticized if it did not at least acknowledge the New York study. If it did not show the results of the New York model, it would need to provide compelling rationale for not doing so, because the New York model serves as such a common yardstick for evaluating mortality following bypass surgery.

## Conclusion

All risk stratification involves the analysis and standardization of rates. Whether it is univariate risk taken over strata, as in direct age standardization, or multivariate risk described by a logistic model, the adjustment of observed rates to those of an external standard is the central concept. The mathematical dimensions are different, but the interpretation is the same. In the multivariate case we use the logit transformation for computational reasons to get to probability. From probability we compute expected cases, and from expected cases we get an estimate of the performance of the local center, risk-adjusted and relative to the standard. Confidence intervals and statistical significance testing can assist in interpretation of the findings, as long as appropriately large samples are considered.

## REFERENCES

1 Hennekens CH, Buring JE. *Epidemiology in Medicine.* Little, Brown, Boston, 1987.

2 Hannan EL, Kilburn H Jr., Racz M, Shields E, Chassin MR. Improving the outcomes of coronary artery bypass surgery in New York State. *JAMA* 1994; **271**: 761–6.

3 Rothman KJ, Boice JD. *Epidemiologic Analysis with a Programmable Calculator.* NIH Publication No. 79–1649, U.S. Department of Health, Washington, D.C., 1979.

4 Rosner, B. *Fundamentals of Biostatistics*, third edition. PWS-Kent, Boston, 1990.

5

# Interpreting risk models

We have covered interpretation of risk stratification results to some degree in Chapters 1 and 4 thus far. We have seen that stratified data and logistic regression coefficients taken from one population can be used to standardize or to predict events in another. These are very powerful tools, and their proper use and interpretation require attention not only to the mechanics of the arithmetic, but also to the issues of bias and underlying population characteristics. In this chapter, we will review some of the familiar interpretation issues briefly, and then will cover some broader concepts related to the depth of the risk inquiry and the presentation of data.

## Population characteristics and their distribution

The importance of comparability between standard populations and local study populations with regard to the distribution and prevalence of risk factors cannot be overstated. Multivariable risk models cannot reasonably compare populations that are grossly different with respect to their underlying risk characteristics. This is because the weighting of risk factor coefficients will be different in populations where risk factors are common than it will be in populations where the risk factors are rare. A risk factor that is rare in a population, even if it is strong, will account for only a small number of events in that population. If the *events* being studied are common, the small number of events attributable to the rare risk factor will also be a small *proportion* of the overall events, and the factor will not look important in that context. But this same risk factor, if it were common in another population, might account for a large proportion of events in that population, since it is, after all, a strong risk factor. Problems would arise if a model developed on a population where a certain risk factor was rare were subsequently applied to another population where the factor was common. In mathematical models, the strength of any risk factor is represented mainly by the size of the factor's associated regression coefficient. If a strong risk factor is rare in a standard population and therefore accounts for only a small proportion of the events in that population, the coefficient associated with the risk factor will be either incorrectly sized or will be associated with so much statistical error that it will be dropped from the model as non-predictive (i.e., not statistically significant). When a model developed on a study sample that had a low prevalence of a particular risk factor is applied to a local population in which the prevalence of a risk factor is high, the predictions will be inaccurate. This is either because the coefficient is improperly sized or because it was never included in the standard model because of low statistical power. When a risk factor is not properly accounted for in a statistical model, as we have seen previously, the model cannot explain population events on the basis of the risk factor, and the model equations will be inaccurate for predicting events in another population where the risk factor is prevalent. The weights attached to regression coefficients for strong risk factors can vary considerably between populations that have large differences in prevalences of the factor. For this reason, comparability of the underlying characteristics of two populations is essential when weighted coefficients from one are to be used to predict events in another. In general, the prevalence of important risk factors should not differ by more than 20 percent between the standard and the local populations. We strongly advocate that reports written about both the development of risk equations and the application of them should show univariate data that describe population risk factor prevalences. Without information on risk factor prevalence, results of risk predictions, and deficiencies in their fit characteristics, are difficult to interpret.

## Bias

Another problem related to populations and their characteristics has to do with differential data ascertainment between populations. If

**Selection bias**
A bias of selection exists when treatment or group assignment is correlated with patient characteristics.

estimates of risk factor occurrence in a population or the association of the risk factors with outcome are non-uniformly ascertained for some reason, a bias is said to be present in the study. *Selection bias* is a notorious bias and can be very difficult to ferret out. Selection bias occurs when population members are selected to a treatment group or other group on the basis of some sort of personal characteristic. The clearest examples of the effects of selection bias occur in efficacy research. If patients with a certain severity of illness routinely seek one treatment over another, the effects of the treatment might be biased by the way patients are selected to the treatment. For example, patients with extremely severe emphysema might seek lung volume reduction surgery more aggressively than patients whose emphysema is less severe – the sicker, more desperate patients might be more willing to take a chance on high-risk surgery than the less severely affected patients. Poor results in the surgical group might be attributable to some extent to their more severe underlying illness, and may not only reflect mortality associated with the surgical procedure. Efficacy-oriented studies deal best with bias through the experimental control of treatment. Control groups and ideally randomization to treatment are needed to separate the effects of the treatment from the underlying problem that brought patients to seek treatment in the first place. Randomized clinical trials, as the strongest research design, can separate treatment effects from any source of bias that depends on patients' characteristics.

In the risk-stratification situation, because of the difference in focus, selection bias causes a different kind of group accrual problem. In risk analysis, as opposed to clinical efficacy research, the primary hypothesis test is aimed not at treatment, but at the population. Where patients are allocated to treatments in efficacy research, they are allocated to populations in risk-stratification studies, and all the patients in a risk-stratification study undergo the same treatment. The presumption in a randomized clinical trial is that a difference in event rate between treatment groups will be a reflection of the quality of a specific treatment. In risk-stratification studies, on the other hand, the presumption is that a difference in the event rate will reflect the quality of care provided to a specific population. So while we worry about selection to treatment in efficacy studies, we worry similarly about selection to population in the risk-stratification situation. Just as patient characteristics that lead patients to seek certain treatments can bias the evaluation of those treatments, so patient characteristics that lead patients to seek care at a particular institution can bias our conclusions about the quality of care provided by that institution. The usual interpretation of a risk-stratification study is that, once differences in population characteristics have been accounted for, differences between expectation and outcome are due to quality of care for the local population. But this assumes that everything that would affect outcome (i.e., everything that would be a risk factor) can be accounted for and measured. We know that this is not always possible in clinical research, so we rely on randomized designs to minimize the likelihood of bias in ascertainment of treatment results. The strongest scientific test for institutional quality of care, which is the usual endpoint of risk stratification, would be randomization of patients into two different clinic populations to see which group had the better outcome. This would be the strongest design for the same reasons why it is so in clinical efficacy research. But as a practical matter, patients cannot be randomized to one population instead of another. Geography, patient preference, insurance coverage, and other issues control institutional population membership. So risk stratification necessarily takes the observational rather than the experimental approach to dealing with the effects of population characteristics on outcome.

As we have seen, selection bias is a systematically different accrual of patients to one group compared to another. Selection bias is perhaps the best known form of bias, but other biases can cause problems as well. *Information bias* occurs when information is collected or reported differently between groups. Interviewer bias is one form of information bias. Interviewer bias occurs when data collected from patients are pursued more aggressively in one group or recorded differently than in another. Recall bias is another form of information bias, where patients with certain illnesses or conditions might recall past exposures differently from patients without such illnesses.

**Information bias**
Information bias occurs when the type or character of information obtained from study members differs systematically because of the study group.

Interviewer bias might affect a risk-stratification study in the following way. If an interviewer or examiner at one institution believed that certain risk factors such as exercise were important in decreasing mortality following coronary bypass surgery, he or she might probe more aggressively into exercise history than an interviewer at another institution who did not consider exercise history during the interview. Even if exercise history was not among the variables required to solve a particular risk model, the increased interviewer probing surrounding it might affect the ascertainment of other related variables, such as smoking history, family history of heart disease, etc. Interviewers can also bias risk factor reporting if they appear to be judgmental. Interviewers who are openly critical of smoking, for example, might cause patients to underreport smoking. Training of interviewers to minimize this type of bias is essential for any risk-stratification program that requires direct interviews with patients or other respondents such as family members.

Recall bias is another important form of information bias. Recall bias refers to the likelihood that a patient or someone responding to an interview on the patient's behalf might have a different probability of recalling previous exposures in one group than another. A classic example of this from the literature on efficacy is that of recall bias in the parents of children with childhood cancers. Parents of children with cancer are much more likely to have spent hours poring over the past, trying to remember any event – a dental radiograph, a spilled can of solvent – that could possibly have some bearing on the current family tragedy.

As with selection bias, information bias causes different kinds of problems for risk-stratification studies than for efficacy/exposure studies. In efficacy studies, the potential for information bias is highest in situations where the outcome is already known (e.g., in case–control studies). In risk-stratification studies, information bias is only a problem when it affects populations differently, since treatment is the same for everyone, and outcome is not known beforehand in prospective study designs. Anything that causes ascertainment of risk factors to be different in the population that serves as the standard than it is in the local population for which risk is being predicted can introduce bias. In a risk-stratification study of health services utilization among patients with pulmonary fibrosis, for example, information about exposure to substances that are potentially damaging to pulmonary tissue might be ascertained very differently in a group of West Virginia coal miners than it would be in a group of Southern California dentists. Both the interviewers' probing and the recall of the patient might be affected by well-described problems of exposure to free silica associated with mining, even though some of the older dentists might have had significant exposure to porcelain dust in dental laboratories over the years. Either group's occupational exposures could lead to pulmonary silicosis (1,2), which can be superimposed on or confused with other types of fibrosis, but the risks in one group are much better known than they are in the other, and that may change the intensity of the work-up and the frequency of the diagnosis between the groups. If occult pulmonary silicosis is a risk factor for increased health services utilization, as we would expect it to be, under-ascertainment of silicosis in the dentists would cause there to be more unexplained utilization in that group.

Ideally, information bias due to prior knowledge of the outcome should not be a problem in risk-stratification studies, which are prospective by design. Bias due to prior knowledge of outcome occurs mainly in chart review studies, when chart reviewers can tell from medical records what the outcome is at the time of risk factor ascertainment. Bias with regard to prior knowledge of outcome is not a major problem unless, as with all other problematic risk-stratification biases, the magnitude or nature of the bias occurs differently in the local population than it does in the population chosen as a standard. That is, if both the standard study and the local study were done using retrospective chart reviews, biases in risk factor ascertainment would be expected to be approximately equal in magnitude and nature between the standard and the local populations. Biased ascertainment does not cause a directional bias in the observed/expected (*O*/*E*) ratio estimate unless it is different in one population than it is in another. Although the potential for such bias can be worrisome, for practical reasons data for many risk-stratification studies need to be collected from hospital charts after the outcome has occurred and is known. Historical cohort designs are quite common in the actual practice of risk stratification. For reasons of efficiency and cost, chart-based risk-stratification studies usually involve a single review of each chart after the patient has been discharged from hospital or has died. It may be extremely difficult for chart reviewers to avoid digging deeper for explanations in cases where the outcome occurs, because of the natural impulse to uncover data that will explain the occurrence of the event. Because of this, some degree of information

**→ TIP 1**

If possible, to avoid bias, chart reviewers should be blinded to outcome.

bias in ascertainment of risk factors is unavoidable in chart-review-based work. Biases due to abstractor knowledge of outcome are subtle and can be very difficult to identify, so the magnitude and direction of such a bias on *O*/*E* ratios may be extremely difficult to estimate. The best way to avoid information bias due to outcome is to collect all the risk factor data before the outcome occurs. Since risk-stratification predictions are based on preintervention risk factors, it is actually possible to do this. Unfortunately, pretreatment risk factor ascertainment would require a labor-intensive two-stage chart review, one for identification of pretreatment risk factors and a second for ascertainment of the outcome. This type of staged review may not be feasible for numerous reasons. When staged review is not possible, steps should be taken to minimize prior knowledge biases, and quality control audits that look specifically for these kinds of differences in risk factor ascertainment associated with known outcome should be undertaken.

How selection or information biases that are internal to populations affect inferences in risk studies depends on several things. As for the *O*/*E* ratio and its interpretation, as long as biases present in one study are of the same direction and magnitude as in the other study, the *O*/*E* ratio should not be biased directionally. A directional bias is one in which the *O*/*E* estimate would be biased either up or down, regardless of the position of the estimate with regard to the null *O*/*E* value. The null *O*/*E* value is 1.0 – no difference between observed and expected. In a study with a downward directional bias, say, in which a large risk factor was over-ascertained in the local population, the expected value for the local will always be higher than it should be and will bias the *O*/*E* ratio downward. Local risk factor overascertainment happens when data abstractors "game the system", say, by fudging instances of complex, high-risk diagnoses. For example, chronic obstructive pulmonary disease (COPD) is a major risk factor for mortality following coronary bypass surgery. COPD is also a complex diagnosis and can be difficult to ascertain from a medical chart. If an abstractor wanted to improve the perceived results of the local institution, he or she might code every patient with a 20-pack-year smoking history as having COPD. This would increase the expected number of deaths in the local population by inflating the prevalence of this important risk factor. Because the expected value, the denominator of the *O*/*E* ratio, would be overly large, the ratio calculated from it would be smaller than it should be, and this would be true no matter whether the institution was actually doing better or worse than expected. If they were doing worse, the amount by which they were over the estimated target would be reduced by the bias. If they were doing better than expected in reality, the bias would make it seem as though they were doing better still. The position of the *O*/*E* ratio with respect to the null value of 1.0 would not matter.

If bias in the populations does not differ materially *between populations*, the effect on the *O*/*E* ratio is not directional. Essentially, bias in ascertainment that is constant between populations is random with respect to the hypothesis test of interest. That is, if misclassification of a certain risk factor, say, smoking history, were the same in the standard population as it was in the local population, the effect on the *O*/*E* ratio would be to bias it toward the null value of 1.0. The amount of unexplained morbidity due to unrecognized smoking would be the same in both populations. Random misclassification between populations would tend to make the populations more alike with respect to the influence of risk factors, by increasing the amount of the event probability that is unexplained. Since the purpose of the *O*/*E* ratio is to test for differences between populations, any bias that makes the populations more alike will reduce the magnitude of the *O*/*E* ratio. This is a bias toward the null, which arises from generalized lack of precision in the estimates.

## Missing data

Beyond the biases that can occur from problems with selection, information and recall are biases that can occur because of missing data. It is not difficult to imagine that significant biases could occur with respect to a single variable if that variable were to be missing in a large proportion of the subjects enrolled in a risk-stratification study. Missing data means incomplete information, and decreased precision for modeling, at best. At worst, data are missing for a reason, because of some sort of bias, and this is known as informative missingness. Any time data are missing because of a correlation between data ascertainment and patient characteristics, the potential for bias exists. Informative missingness is particularly troublesome in follow-up studies, where patients are discharged from care and then re-evaluated at another time. Patients who do not show up for follow-up are almost always those who were unhappy with their treatment or outcome. These are the people we would actually most like to talk to, to find out what kinds of problems they are having and to develop strategies for improving the outcomes for patients like them in the future. Missing data on such people leads us to the false conclusion that everyone is doing well and we underascertain problems in the population as a result. Underascertainment of problems leads to overly optimistic risk estimates.

But what may be less apparent is the fact that the effect of missing data on a single variable can go beyond the effect of that variable alone in the introduction of bias into a sample. Recall that when we solved multivariate models in Chapter 4, we multiplied values for each variable through the logistic regression coefficients in the model. When a variable's value was greater than zero, the value of the predictor was the variable's value multiplied by its corresponding regression coefficient. When the value of the variable was zero, the multiplication caused the value of the term for that variable to go to zero, and the predictor effectively dropped out of the model, which is additive in its accumulation of terms. So what happens when a variable's value is missing? While we might intuitively expect to set the value of a missing variable to zero, so that we could just drop out the term and ignore it, doing that would actually have many undesirable properties. For most continuous variables – age, ejection fraction, etc. – zero values are simply wrong (age) or incompatible with life (ejection fraction). For indicator variables, "not known" is not the same as "not present". It would be an error to say that a person whose gender is unknown defaults to female, or that a person whose diabetes history is unknown is a person without diabetes. So missing values cannot be handled as zeroes, they have to be handled as missing. What happens when we multiply a missing value against a regression coefficient? All the data for that patient, not just the value of the missing variable, are lost. If we only dropped out the coefficient when a value was missing, that would not be right, because that coefficient would have the same interpretation as a zero observation. Zero values for indicator variables, though, indicate that a person does not have a risk factor, *not* that

> **→ TIP 2**
>
> Missing data have a great potential to bias studies. Design studies with completeness of variable ascertainment in mind.

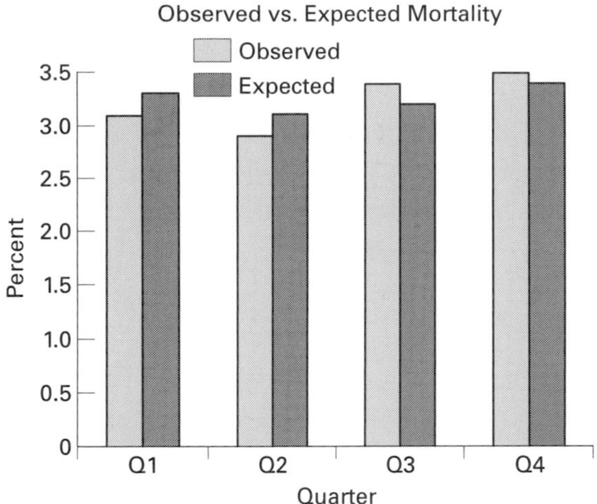


Figure 5.1 Observed and model expected mortality in percent for four hypothetical calendar quarters.

the risk factor simply could not be ascertained. We cannot therefore code missing data the same as not having a risk factor.

Randomly missing data, like randomly misclassified data, will not cause a directional bias in the risk estimates but will only decrease the statistical power of the comparisons by causing the groups to be more alike. Informatively missing data, on the other hand, can cause significant directional biases that may not be reparable at the analysis stage. For this reason, every effort needs to be made to ascertain data as completely as possible, even for the most difficult to evaluate segments of the population. Only data that are important should be collected, but *all* data that are important should be collected.

## Presentation of results

Graphs and tables are very useful for presenting the results of risk-stratification studies. Several approaches are possible, depending on the purpose and target audience of the report. For quarterly or other summary reports that describe a time period, bar graphs can be used to summarize actual and expected events. Figure 5.1 shows one possibility for a bar graph showing the relative frequencies of expected and actual

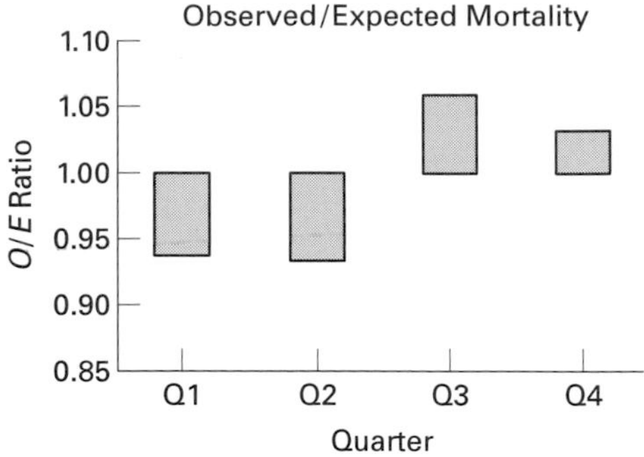


Figure 5.2 **Data shown in Figure 5.1 expressed as *O/E* ratio. When expected is larger than observed, the ratio is less than one. When observed is larger than expected, the ratio is greater than one.**

outcome. Data are arrayed by calendar quarter across the *X*-axis and percent events (in this case mortality) are shown on the *Y*-axis. The light bars are actual mortality, and the dark bars are expected. We see that in the first quarter, the observed mortality is 3.1 percent, while expected is 3.3 percent. For the second, observed is 2.9 percent and expected is 3.12 percent. For the third quarter observed is 3.4 percent while expected is 3.2 percent, and for the fourth quarter observed is 3.5 percent and expected 3.4 percent. In the first two quarters, the program being reviewed is exceeding expectations. For the second two quarters, it is lagging slightly behind. Figure 5.2 shows the same data arrayed as *O/E* ratios. For ratios, 1.0 is the null value, so the bars start from a baseline of 1.0. The first quarter *O/E* ratio is 3.1 observed divided by 3.3 expected, which is equal to 0.939. So the first quarter results indicate that the observed mortality rate is 93.9 percent of the expected – a very good result. The last quarter, in contrast, is 3.5 observed divided by 3.4 expected, for an *O/E* ratio of 1.03. This indicates that the observed mortality is three percent higher than the risk model would have expected. If we wanted to know about the variation associated with each estimate, we might plot 95 percent confidence intervals with the figures. Figure 5.3 shows the same quarterly arrangement of *O/E* ratios from Figure 5.2 plotted with their 95 percent confidence intervals. Confidence interval width is a function of

> **→ TIP 3**
> Plot confidence intervals with point estimates whenever possible.

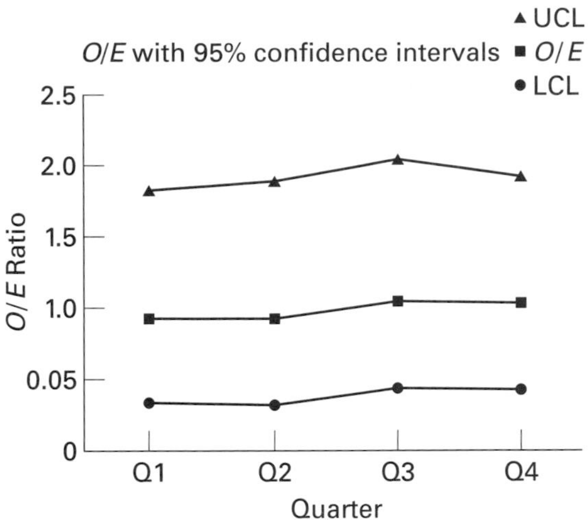


Figure 5.3 Data from Figure 5.2 shown with 95% confidence intervals. Confidence intervals reflect variance associated with sample size $n = 200$ per quarter. Note that the intervals are quite wide even with a relatively large sample. *LCL*, lower confidence limit; *UCL*, upper confidence limit.

the variation in the *O*/*E* ratio and the confidence level (95 percent in this case) chosen. Variation associated with a ratio is a function of the size of the sample. In the example shown in Figure 5.3, we assumed that the sample size was 250 cases per quarter. As we can see, the *O*/*E* ratio point estimates hover around 1.0 across the four time points. The upper interval is well above 1.0 (around 2.0), and the lower interval is well below 1.0 (around 0.35). Confidence intervals at the 95 percent level have the property of excluding the null value ($O/E = 1.0$) when the *O*/*E* ratio is statistically significantly different from the null at the traditional $p < 0.05$ level of alpha error. Therefore, if any of the quarterly observed values were statistically different from their expected values, 1.0 would be excluded from the confidence interval. The confidence intervals also tell us that, based on the sample size and the magnitude of the ratios, we might expect *O*/*E* ratios encountered in future sampling, all things being equal, to vary between about 0.35 and 2.0 95 percent of the time.

In addition to presentation of observed/expected probabilities and ratios, it is sometimes desirable to produce figures of risk that span a

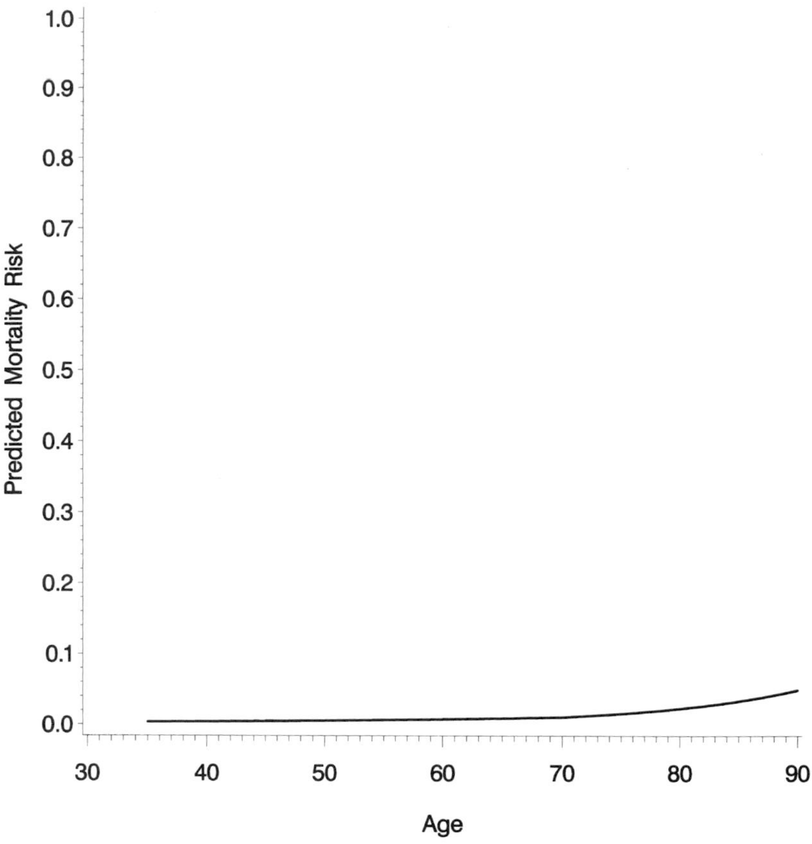


Figure 5.4 Model probability of mortality by age following coronary bypass. Age only without other risk factors.

range of another variable. Figures of this type can help with interpreting the magnitude and scale of risk associated with a continuous variable. Figure 5.4, which also appears as Figure 1.1, shows the relationship between patient age and expected mortality risk for hospital death following coronary bypass surgery. As we can see, risk remains low through the 40s and 50s, begins to increase in the 60s and takes a sharper turn upward beyond 70 years of age. It is possible to plot more than one risk factor at a time, which provides further information about how risk factor variables might interact. Figure 5.5 shows separate probability predictions for male and female patients. Females have a slightly

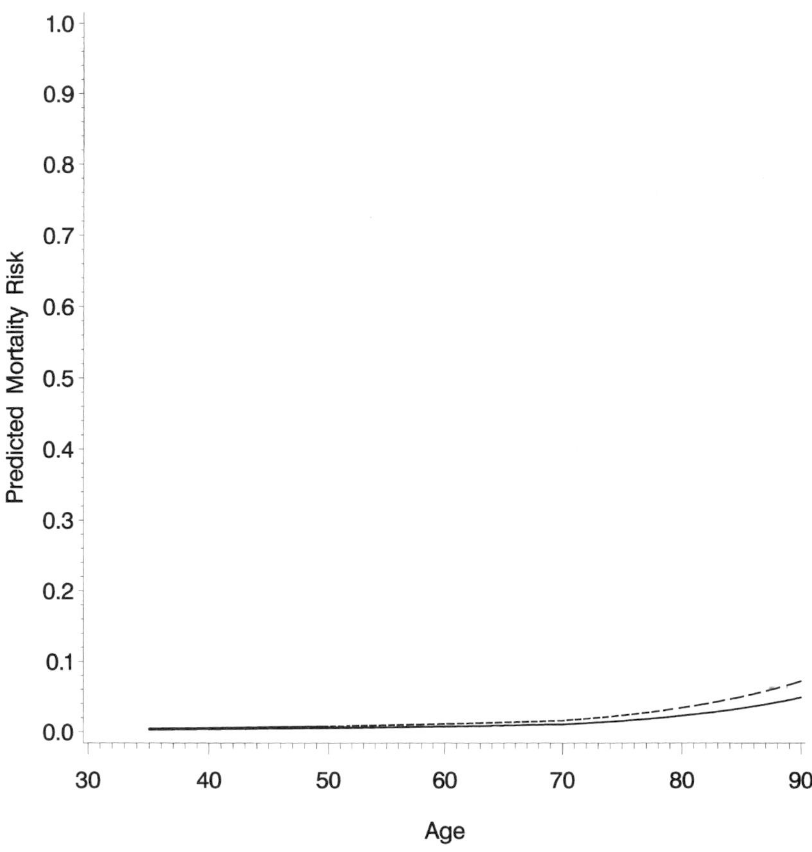


Figure 5.5 Same data as Figure 5.4 but split into males (solid line) versus females (dotted line). Females have slightly higher risk.

higher expected mortality risk than males do for cardiac surgery, and this is reflected in the figure. By age 70 men face an expected risk of approximately one percent, while the risk for females at the same age is approximately 1.5 percent. The lines separate visibly at around age 50, and get further and further apart as the patients get older. Part of this separation is due to legitimately increasing risk with increasing age, and part is due to the exponential form of the model that requires risk to curve upward at an increasing rate. The model that produced these figures does not contain an interaction term – which would be a measure of how rates *change* relative to age. The current model predicts

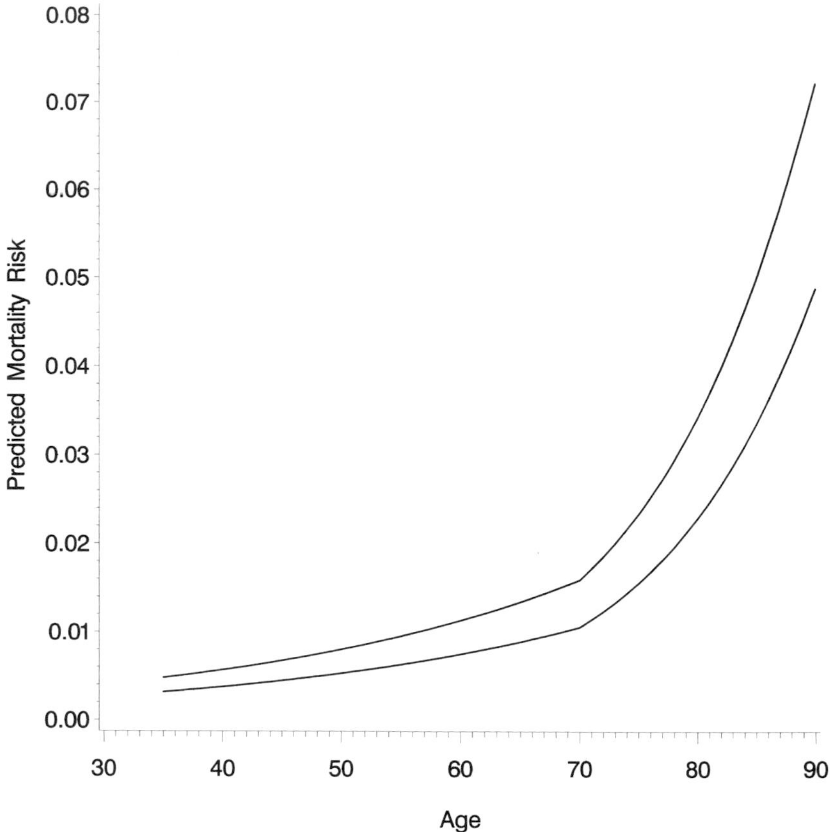


Figure 5.6 Figure 5.5 data not held to 0–1 probability constraints. This figure looks very alarming because of the huge magnification of the scale. Maximum probability in this figure is 8%. Probability figures should always be kept to the entire 0–1 (or 0–100%) range.

a constant exponential rise rather than a differential one that changes in magnitude as the value of age changes.

> **→TIP 4**
>
> Always hold the response axis of probability plots to the full 0–1 range.

While figures can be very helpful in describing and interpreting results, they can also be misleading if attention is not paid to their scale. Figure 5.6 is Figure 5.5 without the predicted risk scale held to its 0–1 constraints. Visually, Figure 5.6 is quite alarming. At a glance, the risk beyond the age of 70 appears to be horrendous, because we tend to expect the scale of a figure to be meaningful. Actually, the maximum value of risk for an 85-year-old female is a little over seven percent, but the scale of the figure only goes to eight percent. For figures that express probabilities, which can only range from zero to one, the entire 0–1 scale should be shown. It is important to confine the probability estimate to its proper context in order to be able to interpret it properly.

## Administrative versus clinical data

In our review of study designs in Chapter 3, we talked about the hierarchy of evidence and the directness of interpretation of cross-sectional, case–control, cohort, clinical trial and risk-stratification studies. We noted that clinical trials were the strongest design, followed by cohort, case–control and finally cross-sectional studies. A hierarchy of evidence exists among risk-stratification studies as well, and the confidence that we are willing to put in their findings is (or should be at any rate) directly proportional to the quality of the evidence they provide. Most of the studies that are published in the medical literature as risk-stratification studies are based on clinical data, and the study design and methods have been subjected to the peer review process. This type of study is the most likely to be applied to local data by academic investigators. However, many other types of risk-stratification studies exist in the community, i.e., those commissioned by insurance companies, posted on the Internet, etc., which are based on administrative data and which have usually not been subjected to peer review. Several versions of administrative-data-based risk-stratification computer routines are available for hospital mainframes and these are often used by institutions to track and risk stratify outcomes, particularly for high-volume high-cost procedures such as coronary bypass. The level of detail and the ability to handle information and selection bias and other risk factor ascertainment problems differ vastly between clinically based and administrative-data-based studies.

Administrative-data-based studies can be appealing at face value for a number of reasons. First of all, the data are readily available from administrative computer systems, which all health-care organizations have. These administrative data contain rudimentary demographics, such as age and gender, and some diagnostic information on co-morbid conditions. Such data are required for clinical billing for Medicare and for many private insurers. The availability of the information in computer systems makes the incremental cost of getting at the data very small compared to the cost of hiring people to go through charts to collect clinical data. Second, uniform administrative data, particularly for patients in the U.S. Medicare system, are widespread and are available for almost every in-patient hospital in the U.S. This makes risk comparisons between huge numbers of health-care organizations possible, at least in principle, and many organizations have published risk estimates for hospitals across the nation that are based on data from Medicare files. The most commonly used source of such data is the Medicare Provider Analysis and Review (MEDPAR) file, which contains data on hospital discharges, principal and secondary diagnoses, and some limited demographic information. MEDPAR data are publicly available, so access to data is a straightforward matter in this case.

Despite wide availability and ease and economy of access, many problems exist with attempts to stratify risk on the basis of administrative data. One major problem with use of administrative data for risk stratification is the fact that patients can have many physiological abnormalities that influence their risk but which would not be classified as diagnoses. A low left ventricular ejection fraction (EF), for example, is known to increase the risk of in-hospital mortality following coronary bypass surgery, but low EF is not a diagnosis, and no administrative code for low EF exists. Innumerable such examples are present in nearly every field of medicine, and this problem poses an inherent limitation that cannot be overcome in large administrative databases as they exist currently. The lack of detail makes it impossible for administrative database studies to classify risk as accurately as clinical variable models can. Furthermore, although databases like the MEDPAR file contain information on co-morbid conditions, it is usually not possible to tell from administrative data whether a co-morbid illness existed prior to a medical intervention (such as surgery) or whether it arose as a complication some time after the intervention but during the episode of care (3). Even in circumstances where dates of service can be used to discriminate between pre-existing co-morbidities and complications of treatment, the classification system by which the co-morbid diagnoses are recorded can be insensitive to the degree of co-morbid illness. MEDPAR uses the International Classification of Diseases 9th revision (ICD-9) to classify co-morbid conditions, and insensitivity in the classification codes may affect the accuracy of risk estimation. For example, ICD-9 code 410.9, acute myocardial infarction within the past eight days, cannot discriminate between a week-old and an hour-old myocardial infarction, even though these have dramatically different impacts on the risk of mortality following coronary bypass surgery (4).

In addition to the problem of low sensitivity and relatively coarse stratification of risk due to limited detail in administrative databases is the problem of bias in the data. Administrative data are collected for billing purposes, not for clinical research. Reimbursement is tied to principal disease coding, and this relationship always carries with it the risk of distortion with respect to the main clinical problem (5). How data are coded for primary and secondary diagnoses, and what variables are collected may vary within and between institutions because of differences in requirements of payers. Institutional culture, geographical region and range of services provided may all affect coding, and can be potential sources of intractable bias. Administrative database studies cannot approach the level of detail available in clinical-variable-based risk studies, and are considered to be weak designs from a quality of inference standpoint.

## Some guidelines for application and interpretation of the methods

A reality of measuring quality of care is that risk factor differences do exist between populations, and these differences interfere with the interpretation of outcome. If risk factors did not differ among populations after all, risk stratification would not need to exist as a field of study. Risk stratification was developed to deal with inhomogeneities in risk factor distribution between populations, by taking differences in population risk factor prevalences into account. As we mentioned in Chapter 4, the traditional interpretation of a standardized population is that differences between the observed and the expected values cannot be attributed to the risk factors that have been measured. They must be attributed to something else. That is, the effects of properly accounted for risk factors have been "adjusted out" of differences between populations. But, as we have also pointed out at length, sometimes differences between populations

**Table 5.1** Guidelines for applying published risk data to a local population

**These guidelines apply to both the standard and the local population:**
**A risk-stratification study is practical if:**

- The disease being treated is the same.
- The treatment for the disease is essentially the same.
- The case and variable definitions are the same.
- The methods for ascertainment of variables and cases are the same.
- The prevalence of the risk factors is roughly the same.
- The studies have at least 100 subjects each if the event rate is ten percent or greater, or at least 250 cases if the event rate is less than ten percent.

**This applies to the standard only:**

- Well-known risk factors should not have less than a two percent prevalence.

are so great that use of one population to standardize or make predictions about another is impossible. The important question is "when does the heterogeneity between two populations, that we would like to adjust out of a comparison, become too big to deal with?" Statistical techniques are available to assist in making formal assessments to some extent, but some simple rules of thumb will suffice most of the time. Table 5.1 is a list of guidelines for when a risk-stratification study can reasonably be undertaken. The disease being treated has to be the same. For example, a local study of mortality risk following coronary bypass surgery should use equations from a standard population of coronary bypass patients, not, say, from a cardiac valve study, which would measure risk for a different clinical problem. Severity of disease can and will vary – that is what the risk factors describe. The treatment has to be principally the same. For example, angioplasty should not be compared to coronary bypass using risk stratification, because the indications for treatment are likely to be too different. Comparison of treatment efficacy is the domain of traditional clinical research – preferably clinical trials – not risk stratification. Case and variable definitions, ascertainment and accounting for important missing data should be comparable between the standard and the

**Table 5.2** Contraindications to application of published risk data to a local population

**A risk-stratification study should not be undertaken if:**

- The prevalence of major risk factors differs by more than 20 percent between the populations.
- Unmeasured population characteristics – such as socioeconomic status – are likely to be very different.
- Events are extremely rare (<1%).

local population. Underlying prevalences of risk factors should be roughly the same, and this should be confirmed by frequency statistics on both populations if at all possible. In the best of circumstances, published risk-stratification standard equations will have been developed on thousands, or tens of thousands of patients. The larger the sample size, in general, the greater the statistical power to tease out the small effects of the many variables whose aggregate effect may result in a significant overall risk. Missing the importance of many small effects may increase the amount of model uncertainty (model error), and consequently the proportion of events that are unexplained, dramatically. Huge risk-stratification studies for widely applied treatments are fairly common, and should be used preferentially when they are compatible with a local research question.

Table 5.2 lists potential contraindications to using one population to standardize another. A rule of thumb is that prevalences for major risk factors should not differ by more than 20 percent between the populations. More than that is likely to cause the coefficient weighting to be inappropriate. Unmeasured population characteristics should be considered as well. Many population characteristics may affect underlying risk, and many of them will not have been accounted for in standard population models. For example, a study of risk of asthma hospitalization done in the pristine air and lifestyle environs of a group of people living in rural Utah may not be very applicable to a population that lives with the air quality of inner-city Los Angeles. Since ground-level ozone is a known risk factor for asthma hospitalization, use of a standard from central Utah, where ozone alerts are unheard of, would miss a major risk factor for the Los Angeles population, where ozone alerts can be a weekly occurrence. Risk-stratification studies attempt to adjust away population differences and attribute remaining differences between observed and expected events to quality of care. It would be a stretch indeed to say that, on the basis of a standard study performed in Utah, increased asthma hospitalizations in Los Angeles was due to lower quality medical care in the Los Angeles area.

Finally, time lag between the standard study and the local study should not be excessive given the process of care milieu for the particular problem under study. In some areas of medicine, where the standard of care has not changed much recently, a time lag of 10–15 years from standard to local study may not be too much. In other areas where the standard of care has evolved rapidly or many new treatments have been introduced, two to five years may be too long. The judgment about how much lag between studies is too much needs to be based on a solid familiarity with the pertinent literature over the previous ten years at a minimum.

## Conclusion

No matter how strong the design or how good the data, a degree of uncertainty will always surround the process of predicting outcome from pretreatment variables. A certain amount of unexplained variation is present in biological systems. This is a fact of life. Far too many unknown influences on outcome are present in nature for us to be able to measure all of them, and some of them are so rare that they cannot be used to produce reliable predictions about the future. Explaining an event after the fact and predicting it beforehand are entirely different processes, and risk stratification is not intended to be a tool for explanation. Explanation of clinical outcomes after the fact is best handled through an institutional morbidity and mortality review process. Risk stratification is a useful tool for producing expectations about the *average* likely experience of a population. The models do not do a good job of predicting extreme or unusual events, and they are not intended to serve this purpose. Post-hoc review is much more useful than risk stratification for identifying specific variances from standards of care and for reviewing extreme outlier cases. Risk stratification is useless for predicting outliers, which are by definition outside of the normal predicted range.

If they are used and interpreted carefully, risk-stratification models can help to sharpen our expectations about the future and can assist us in making inferences about quality of care. Investigators and institutions must recognize, however, that many other factors besides *O/E* ratios contribute to the evaluation of quality of care, and the entire clinical milieu should be considered in the assessment of health-care quality.

## REFERENCES


1 Loewen GM, Weiner D, McMahan J. Pneumoconiosis in an elderly dentist. *Chest* 1988; **93**: 1312–13.

2 DeVuyst P, VandeWeyer R, DeCoster A, Marchandise FX, Dumortier P, Ketelbant P, Jedwab J, Yernault JC. Dental technician's pneumoconiosis. A report of two cases. *Am Rev Respir Dis* 1986; **133**: 316–20.

3 Green J, Wintfeld N. How accurate are hospital discharge data for evaluating effectiveness of care? *Med Care* 1993; **31**: 719–31.

4 Hannan EL, Racz MJ, Jollis JG, Peterson ED. Using Medicare claims data to assess provider quality for CABG surgery: does it work well enough? *Health Serv Res* 1997; **31**: 659–78.

5 Anderson C. Measuring what works in health care. News and Comment. *Science* 1994; **263**: 1080–2.

6

# Advanced issues

Although risk-stratification studies or reasonable approximations to them are available in the literature for a wide variety of medical and surgical problems, it is often the case that an acceptable match for a particular problem cannot be found. In this circumstance, the investigator is left with little choice but to compute risk estimates from his or her own data from the ground up. Although this has the potential to be a quagmire, with exercise of reasonable caution, careful attention to assumptions and, when necessary, expert statistical assistance, doing risk-stratification studies from scratch can be both useful and enlightening. Of no small importance also is the fact that such studies can be published, so that where the literature is bereft of pertinent work, there is the potential for benefit both to the investigators and to the overall advancement of the science in that area. If no good studies meeting the criteria we described in Chapter 3 are to be found, investigators are encouraged to consider pursuing an original risk analysis. In contrast with the calculator- or spreadsheet-level computations we have done thus far, a good quality statistical software package is essential for the actual construction of risk models. Our personal favorite is SAS, the Statistical Analysis System, but others are available. All of the examples that follow are from SAS programs. The major programs are similar in their approaches to these problems.

## Types of studies

As we mentioned in Chapter 3, where we described the evaluation of published studies, the first thing to be determined during the contemplation of any original research is the study question. The type of study required for an appropriate risk analysis depends on the question to be answered. Many different study designs can be employed, and sometimes more than one can be used for a particular situation. Usually, however, one particular design will stand out as being stronger than the other candidates, and the design with the strongest inferential properties is the most desirable. In practice, most risk-stratification studies that are intentionally undertaken as risk studies are observational. It is uncommon, although not impossible by any means, to structure a risk-stratification study as a clinical trial. Clinical trials are extremely resource-intensive (expensive), and are usually undertaken to answer a specific question about the effectiveness of a particular treatment.

In Chapter 3 we described several different study types, and we pointed out that the majority of risk data are available from cohort studies, case–control studies, risk studies, and cross-sectional studies. Cohort studies start with risk factors and look forward in time to the onset of disease in the study sample. The statistics provided by cohort studies are incidence statistics. Case–control studies are prevalence studies that look backward in time from prevalent diseased and non-diseased groups to risk factor sets that are statistically associated with the disease. Risk-stratification studies are usually a hybrid – they are studies of cumulative incidence over a period that is handled mathematically as a period prevalence.

Prospective cohort designs are usually the strongest observational designs, because they quantify the rate at which disease arises in a study group conditional on risk factors. The major exception to this is where diseases or events are rare, under which circumstances case–control studies are usually preferable. Since studies used for risk stratification are intended to serve as some sort of standard, the main determinant in the choice of design is usually what kind of outcome is to be compared to the standard. In the case of mortality following coronary bypass surgery, since the endpoint always occurs after surgery, the prospective (cohort) design is usually implied. That is not to say that a post hoc review of risk factors among patients who died versus those who survived would not be useful – often case–control studies of this type can be much more powerful for identifying risk factors, since in-hospital mortality following bypass surgery is a relatively rare event. But ultimately, in studying the risk of mortality associated with bypass surgery, it will be desirable to know something about the rate of death that is to be expected based on certain risk factor profiles. Case–control studies, because they select study members on the basis of outcome, cannot by definition tell us anything about the rate at which the outcome arises in the population. Model regression coefficients derived from case–control studies, where case subjects are chosen on the basis of having experienced the outcome, will not be weighted appropriately for estimating outcome probability when applied prospectively to populations where the events are rare. Case–control studies represent a first step, in that risk factors identified in these studies can be applied prospectively in cohort studies to determine their relationship to incidence.

## Design issues

**→ TIP 1**

A literature review is always the first step in development of a *de novo* risk-stratification study.

A literature review is always the first step in undertaking an original risk study. Even if there are no formal risk-stratification studies or other appropriately informative prospective studies in the literature, something (usually many things) will have been written about the problem, and those papers will have attempted to explain the problem's occurrence in relation to some associated risk factor or factors. We do not advocate using the risk-stratification approach for problems that have not been well reported in the literature. The epidemiology of the problem needs to have been pretty well worked out previously, and if that has not been done it is a job for epidemiologists, not risk stratifiers. The most appropriate time to take on an original risk-stratification project is when the problem is well described and the risk factors are generally known, but no *standards* for risk in the particular area are available. Risk stratification is about standardization among study groups. It is not intended to replace population-based epidemiology.

The literature can also be very helpful in the construction of an appropriate case definition for the study, since this will influence the relative frequency of the outcome and will be a central determinant in the ability of other investigators to compare their own data to the findings of the study. When the outcome is death in hospital, as with our coronary bypass example, the case definition is straightforward. Death is easy to ascertain in most cases, and it is rare that people recover from it. In many disease outcomes, however, it will be necessary to define an outcome as an arbitrary threshold in some continuous or ordinal measure (say, the prothrombin time required to classify someone as having a coagulopathy). In other cases, the time of ascertainment may be critical, because some diseases get better with time and/or treatment. Too short a follow-up and the disease may not have been expressed; too long and it may have come and gone.

Another consideration in establishing a case definition is the problem of competing risks. Competing risks mainly influence the *ascertainment* of cases, but can have some effect on case definition as well. Initially, an investigator might wish to predict the probability that someone will contract a disease or a particular complication, and then might like to go on to predict the probability of mortality as well. Good methods for predicting the probabilities of disease and subsequent mortality *all in one model* do not exist at present. Predicting repeat episodes of a disease or post-treatment complication is also fraught with methodological problems. In general, modeling techniques are good for one event and one event only per model, and even then competing risks can lead to difficulties in interpretation of the results. Heart valve replacements are a good example (1). People who require heart valve replacement usually have other forms of heart disease and tend to be older than the general population. Both of these characteristics predispose heart valve patients – even those treated successfully – to increased risk of mortality. One of the determinants of a successful heart valve operation is freedom from re-operation over time. But a patient who dies with a functioning valve did not have a valve failure and is considered a "success" with regard to freedom from re-operation in terms of outcome coding. Despite freedom from re-operation, however, this patient should not be said to have had a good outcome. In situations such as long-term heart valve function, where the events are studied in populations with a high risk of mortality, freedom from re-operation statistics may grossly under-represent the favorable outcome rate. This is not only a problem for long-term outcomes. Patients who die on the operating table also can not be evaluated for outcomes such as valve failure. Any competing event that would interfere with our ability to evaluate outcome affects

consumption of blood products, are highly influential predictors of neurological outcome (2–9). Unfortunately, these intra-operative variables are also useless to us for predicting how patients will do *before* we operate on them, because many factors that we cannot know in advance may affect clamp time, blood product usage, etc. If we would like to use risk data to counsel a patient on the likelihood that paralysis will occur following surgery, we can consider variables such as the patient's age and gender, extent of disease, and concurrent medical illnesses. But we cannot know prior to surgery how long the cross-clamp will need to be in place, how many units of packed red blood cells will need to be transfused, etc. While these variables are largely correlated with disease extent, they do vary considerably within individuals with similar disease, because of anatomical considerations and other factors that are specific to each patient. Therefore, at least initially, we need models that can predict risk on the basis of *preoperative* variables – risk that can be described before we know what the intra-operative variables are likely to do.

This is not to say that intra-operative variables are unimportant for preoperative risk-stratification studies. We have found it to be true in our experience that improvements in operative technique reduce the morbidity and mortality associated with various types of operations, and that the reduction in untoward events in turn changes the weights of the preoperative predictor variable coefficients. This causes us to have different risk models over time, without any changes in the predictor variables. Even in models with the exact same variable sets, the risk factor weights change over time as improvements in technique produce better results. Unmeasured process-of-care variables can influence the measured baseline risk variables as the process changes and improvements in care come about. In the early days of aortic surgery, the most extensive thoracoabdominal (Crawford extent 2, or TAAAII) aneurysms carried a risk of neurological deficit of 31–33 percent (10), because of the long clamp times and the complete cessation of blood flow to the spinal cord. In more recent years we have discovered that by using pump perfusion to the distal aorta and decompressing the spinal cord compartment by cerebrospinal fluid drainage, we can reduce the risk of paraplegia in these same extensive aneurysms, to between 5 and 12 percent (2–9). If we had estimated the risk of postoperative paraplegia for a person with a TAAAII aneurysm in 1985, without considering any intra-operative variables, we would have pegged the risk at about 25 percent. Today, for a similar patient (or even the exact same patient considered at a different time), we would estimate it to be less than half that. The preoperative risk factor – TAAAII aneurysm – has not changed, but our expectation with regard to its influence on risk has changed dramatically. The change in intra-operative technique, even though we have not tried to model it in this simple example, is responsible for the difference. Because of advances in medical care, it is useful to re-consider risk factor studies periodically. The risk factors themselves are unlikely to have changed, but the magnitude of risk that we would predict from them might well have.

> **➔ TIP 3**
>
> Because of rapid progress in the treatment of some conditions, risk models should be re-evaluated periodically to determine their ongoing appropriateness for prediction.

Another type of very strong predictor that should generally not be used in risk-stratification models is *intercurrent treatment* (i.e., not the treatment that defines the group). Such treatments are not actually patient characteristics, but are used by some investigators on occasion to act as a surrogate for patient characteristics. The problem with using them for this purpose is that different centers may use particular treatments for different indications, or for the same indication with different thresholds of medical necessity. Use of endotracheal intubation to predict increased length of stay in the intensive care unit (ICU) among neonates with respiratory tract infections would be an example. Different indications for intubation may exist from one center to another, and early intubation may actually prolong the hospital course in certain circumstances for a given severity of illness. Weaning protocols, increased infection risk, etc. may increase the time spent in ICU for babies who are intubated versus babies who are not intubated, even if the babies are equally sick. So use of intubation itself as a risk factor for increased ICU stay may not tell us anything about the underlying disease, only the process of care that is keeping the babies in ICU. If the goal of risk stratification is to highlight differences in quality of care, it would be a mistake to use process-of-care variables in a risk model to describe severity of illness.

Numerous intellectual considerations apply to model construction, beyond the fairly blunt standard of high statistical explanatory power, and we encourage investigators to give careful consideration to the variables they are evaluating. It is also extremely worthwhile to read as much as possible about the topic beforehand. Finally, when the research question is identified, the literature review is done, the study design is worked out, the potential predictor variables are identified, the case definition is established and ascertainment protocols are in place, our attention can turn to data collection.

## Collecting data

We covered the mechanics of this with regard to the use of published study comparisons in Chapter 2, and not much is different in terms of the actual process of collecting, performing quality control on and storing data. What is different is that if a risk model is not available from the literature to specify the data elements needed to solve a specific equation, then the investigators are left with the responsibility of deciding what data to collect. This is the reason why the literature review and determination of study type are necessary early in the process. The literature provides a background for deciding what risk factors to include. Potential risk factors reported in the literature should all be considered for inclusion in a *de novo* risk study, and the inclusion or exclusion of each one in the new study should be justified. Even in circumstances where the investigators think previously described risk factors are unimportant, many people working in the field may have a different view, and lack of adequate justification for ignoring certain risk factors may be a cause of vociferous criticism later on.

In addition to deciding what risk factors to include, data on potentially confounding variables should be included as well. In risk-stratification studies, where we are usually looking for the overall effects of risk factor constellations on outcome, rather than trying to isolate the effect of one particular predictor variable, it may seem a bit odd to characterize certain variables as confounders. We usually think of confounding variables as being associated with both a major risk factor and an outcome, in that they interfere with the inferences we would make about the main variable of interest. This occurs because the confounding variable is correlated with the main predictor variable *with respect to prediction of the outcome*, in some significant way. But in the absence of a singular risk factor of importance, we might be tempted to think of confounders not as confounders, but just as additional contributors to the explanation of variance that are useful to us in making predictions. After all, any variable, regardless of how it affects the multivariate coefficients associated with other risk factors, improves prediction if it decreases unexplained variance. But there are, in fact, variables that confound risk studies. In the context of risk prediction, we think of confounders not so much in terms of the way they interact with other risk factor variables, but in terms of how they affect the inferences that can be drawn from a risk-stratification study. It is quite important, when designing studies, to think of these things in order to avoid having problems with generalizability later on.

In the New York State model of coronary bypass mortality, for example, missing ejection fraction (EF) was identified as an independent risk factor. This was captured by creating an indicator variable that had the value 1 when EF could not be ascertained and 0 when it could. At first, including a separate indicator variable in a prediction model that denotes a missing data value might seem like an odd thing to do. If it's missing, we can't get it and we just don't worry about collecting it, right? Not necessarily. Missing data that are missing at random are not usually troublesome. They will decrease the power of our inferences somewhat, but will not affect model validity. On the other hand, data that are missing otherwise than at random (i.e., for a reason), which are known as informatively missing data, are a different problem entirely. Chapters 3 and 5 deal with missing data and the effect of informative missingness on inferences from published risk-stratification studies. To use the ejection fraction example, EF might be missing because a patient did not have EF measurements made at cardiac catheterization. This might be because an emergency developed in the cardiac catheterization laboratory and the patient had to be taken to emergency surgery. Whatever the reason, as a real-life example, missing EF data was found in the New York model to be a significant predictor of hospital mortality. But here is the greatest problem. Because of the way logistic regression analysis works, any data element that has a missing value throws out an entire patient record, so that none of the data for that particular patient can be used. If missing EF data had just been ignored in the New York model, all the patients with missing values would have been dropped from the study, and the significant explanatory value of a missed EF would have been lost from the model. In a more general sense, any special properties that belong to a category of patients who have chronically missing data of a particular type will be lost to the risk model. Everyone with missing data is excluded from the analysis. Problems with missing data are for risk factors what problems with case ascertainment are for outcomes. Complete data in all arenas are essential for good estimates.

## Univariate analysis

> **→ TIP 4**
>
> Univariate analysis is an important first step in getting to understand relationships in the data. It should not be overlooked or rushed.

Once data have been collected, edited, subjected to quality control audits, and so on, the first step in the analysis is to compute some descriptive statistics. For continuous variables, such as age, univariate statistics such as mean and standard deviation are a first step. It is often useful to look at frequency histograms that show the general distribution of the data. Large departures from normality of distribution can cause problems with inferences made from data. See Rosner (10) for a discussion of normality and parametric statistics. Simple frequency tables are useful descriptive statistics for dichotomous or ordinal data. A first look at dependence of outcome on the various risk factors should also be undertaken early in the game, because these simple statistics can be very helpful in interpreting the results of multivariate statistical models later on.

For dichotomous predictor variables, $2 \times 2$ contingency tables are appropriate. Notation for contingency tables is row-by-column, so a $2 \times 2$ table has two rows and two columns, a $3 \times 2$ has three rows and two columns, and so on. Rows are the horizontal dimension of the table, columns the vertical.

Table 6.1 shows an example of a $2 \times 2$ table. This table shows data from our study of the effects of risk factors on the likelihood of a postoperative paraplegia or paraparesis (neurological deficit) following repair of the thoracoabdominal aorta. We are interested here in the influence of acute aortic dissection, a previously described risk factor, on postoperative neurological outcome. In this table, the rows represent the presence or absence of the outcome (neurological deficit), and the columns represent the risk factor grouping (acute aortic dissection or not).

**Table 6.1** Contingency table analysis of neurological deficit by acute aortic dissection. Computation of odds ratio is shown

| | Acute Dissection | No Dissection | |
|---|---|---|---|
| Neurological Deficit | 4 (12.1%) | 27 (5.2%) | 31 |
| No Neurological Deficit | 29 | 496 | 525 |
| | 33 | 523 | 556 |

Odds in dissection group = 4/29 = 0.1379
Odds in no-dissection group = 27/496 = 0.0544
Odds ratio = 0.1379/0.0544 = 2.53

In the dissection group, we see that four patients of 33, or 12.1 percent, had postsurgical neurological deficit. In the non-dissecting group, we see that 27 of 523, or 5.2 percent, developed neurological deficits. Percent, as we recall from Chapter 1, is a *relative* frequency. The numbers four, 27, 33 and 523 are known as the *cell frequencies*, the numbers 31 and 525 are the *row marginal totals*, and the numbers 33 and 523 are the *column marginal totals*. The number 556 is the *grand total* for the table.

In addition to the simple frequencies and relative frequencies we can compute cell by cell, some measure of the magnitude of the association, such as the odds ratio, is of interest. The odds ratio quantifies the strength of the association between the risk factor and the disease outcome by comparing the odds of having the risk factor for people who have the disease to the odds of having the risk factor in the group that do not have the disease. As its name implies, the odds ratio is the ratio of the odds between two groups. In this case, it is the odds of developing a postsurgical neurological deficit in the acute dissection group divided by the odds of developing a neurological deficit in the non-dissection group. We saw in Chapter 1 that while probability is captured by relative frequency, odds are described by likelihood of an event against likelihood of a non-event. The computations for the odds ratio estimate are shown in the footnote to Table 6.1. In this example, the odds of developing a neurological deficit in the acute dissection group are 4:29 (or 7.25:1 against, using the reduced fraction and conventional gambler's odds notation). In the non-acute-dissection group, odds of neurological deficit are 27:496 (or roughly 18:1 against). Intuitively, we see that 18:1 is somewhat less than half the odds of 7:1, and in fact our calculation shows that the odds ratio is 2.53. We interpret this to mean that the likelihood of a neurological deficit following aortic surgery is roughly two and a half times (2.53 times) greater for patients with acute aortic dissections than for patients without. In general, an odds ratio greater than two is considered to represent a large or important association. However, the odds ratio, like any mathematical estimate based on biological data, is subject to a certain amount of variation. The importance of the variation for statistical significance depends on sample size, the frequency of events, and the magnitude of the association. Significance testing and confidence intervals for the odds ratio both provide useful information about the relationship between the observed odds ratio and chance. One of the most familiar significance tests for contingency table data, and the one on which most confidence interval calculations are based, is the chi square.

The chi square, despite its wide use and consequent great familiarity to readers, is actually an approximation to the Fisher's exact test. The Fisher's test is difficult to compute, and until fairly recently was not practical for large samples. Fast, high-capacity personal computers have changed that, so the Fisher's exact can be computed for nearly any sample at present. The chi square does have some nice generalizations beyond $3 \times 3$, where Fisher's does not apply. Chi square is a test that compares the observed values in a contingency table with values that would be expected to exist in the same table if no relationship between rows and columns were present. Table 6.2 shows the computation of expected values for the chi-square test. To compute expected values for each cell the cell's row margin and column margin are multiplied, and that product is divided by the total sample size. So for the cell in the upper left hand corner, 33 (column margin) is multiplied by 31

**Table 6.2** Application of the chi-square test to contingency table data

Computation of expected values

| | Acute Dissection | No Dissection | |
|---|---|---|---|
| Neurological Deficit | $\frac{33 \times 31}{556}$ | $\frac{523 \times 31}{556}$ | 31 |
| No Neurological Deficit | $\frac{33 \times 525}{556}$ | $\frac{523 \times 525}{556}$ | 525 |
| | 33 | 523 | 556 |

Table of expected values for chi square
Expected values

| | Acute Dissection | No Dissection | |
|---|---|---|---|
| Neurological Deficit | 1.84 | 29.16 | 31 |
| No Neurological Deficit | 31.16 | 493.83 | 525 |
| | 33 | 523 | 556 |

$$\text{Chi square} = \frac{(4-1.84)^2}{1.84} + \frac{(27-29.16)^2}{29.16} + \frac{(29-31.13)^2}{31.13} + \frac{(496-493.83)^2}{493.83} = 2.85$$

$p$ for chi square = 0.091

(row margin), and the product is divided by 556 (grand total). This gives a value of 1.84 neurological deficits that would be expected in the acute aortic dissection population *if acute dissection were* *<u>not</u>* *a risk factor for neurological deficit.* So the null hypothesis for a chi-square test is that no relationship is present between the risk factor and the disease.

The actual test is quite simple. Once the expected values have been computed, each cell's expected value is subtracted from its observed value, and the difference is squared. The cell quantities produced are

**Table 6.3** SAS code for producing an automated analysis of data in Tables 6.1 and 6.2

```
data tab6_3;
input ppe2 acute2 wt;
cards;
1 1 4
1 2 27
2 1 29
2 2 496
;
run;
proc freq;tables ppe2*acute2 / exact;
weight wt;
run;
```

then divided by each cell's expected value, and the sum of the four dividends is taken. This sum follows a chi-square distribution with one degree of freedom, so the $p$ value associated with the observed table can be looked up in a chi-square table. The computations are shown in Table 6.2. We see that the $p$ value is 0.091, which would not lead us to reject the null hypothesis of no relationship in this example at the traditional alpha error rate of $p<0.05$. The larger the differences between the observed table and the expected, the larger the squared differences will be relative to the expected cell sizes, and the more unlikely it is that the observed table will have occurred by chance. Large values of the chi-square quantile translate to small $p$ values.

The chi-square test is not appropriate where *expected* cell sizes are less than five. Most statistics programs will issue a warning when this is the case, and the Fisher's exact test should always be used under these circumstances. The Fisher's exact test requires a large series enumeration of possible tables or a recursive formula, and it is very annoying to compute, so we will not go through it here. Interested readers are referred to Rosner (10) or another suitable introductory statistics text for an explanation of the computations. Table 6.3 shows the SAS code for generating Table 6.1, with the chi-square and the Fisher's exact $p$

values. The SAS output is shown in Table 6.4. The Fisher's $p$ value is 0.103 – still fairly close to the chi square even with the low expected cell problem.

For ordinal risk factor variables with a dichotomous outcome, say, occurrence of postoperative neurological deficit following aortic surgery by quartile of age, a $2 \times N$ contingency table analysis is appropriate, where $N =$ the number of categories in the scale. It is important to keep in mind that most programs will sort ordinal data numerically or alphabetically, and this, depending how variable categories are labeled, may or may not be desirable. For example, if a variable's possible values are <60, 60–67, 68–72, >72, most programs will consider the < and > signs to be character variables and will put the lowest purely numerical value first in the sort. So the sort order in a contingency table analysis would be 60–67, 68–72, <60, >72. Table 6.5 shows the default sort in a SAS program. If the hypothesis is that a linear association exists between the ordinal predictor variable and the outcome, it is not acceptable for the program to sort and to change the order of the ordinal variable. When order is important, the most direct solution is simply to re-code the variables 1, 2, 3, 4 for <60, 60–67, 68–72 and >72, and then the program will order them correctly. Something as trivial seeming as how values are labeled can be extremely important for interpreting ordinal-variable statistics. The conventional chi square, as a measure of general association between rows and columns, will not be affected by order. But tests for linear hypotheses, such as the chi square for trend, will be wrong if the table is set up incorrectly.

The same small-expected cell-size rules that applied to $2 \times 2$ tables also apply to larger ones. Unfortunately, however, Fisher's exact test is difficult to generalize beyond $3 \times 3$, so it may not be possible to compute a valid test of statistical association if expected cell sizes are small. Still, in many programs the chi-square statistic may be the only significance test available for any table beyond $3 \times 3$. One of the ways to deal with this problem is to reduce the number of categories. It is usually possible to collapse table strata together to increase the cell sizes when small expected sizes are a problem. This procedure has the dual benefit of both decreasing the table dimensions and increasing the size of the expected values in each cell.

**Table 6.4** SAS printout produced by program in Table 6.3. Note that the chi-square quantile and p value are identical to those computed in Table 6.2

```
                    The SAS System     10:15 Wednesday, September 29, 1999

                TABLE OF PPE2 BY ACUTE2

          PPE2      ACUTE2

          Frequency|
          Percent  |
          Row Pct  |
          Col Pct  |       1|       2|  Total
          ---------+--------+--------+
                 1 |      4 |     27 |     31
                   |   0.72 |   4.86 |   5.58
                   |  12.90 |  87.10 |
                   |  12.12 |   5.16 |
          ---------+--------+--------+
                 2 |     29 |    496 |    525
                   |   5.22 |  89.21 |  94.42
                   |   5.52 |  94.48 |
                   |  87.88 |  94.84 |
          ---------+--------+--------+
          Total         33      523      556
                      5.94    94.06   100.00


        STATISTICS FOR TABLE OF PPE2 BY ACUTE2

Statistic                        DF       Value        Prob
------------------------------------------------------------
Chi-Square                        1       2.855       0.091
Likelihood Ratio Chi-Square       1       2.219       0.136
Continuity Adj. Chi-Square        1       1.686       0.194
Mantel-Haenszel Chi-Square        1       2.850       0.091
Fisher's Exact Test (Left)                            0.970
                    (Right)                           0.103
                    (2-Tail)                          0.103
Phi Coefficient                           0.072
Contingency Coefficient                   0.071
Cramer's V                                0.072

Sample Size = 556
WARNING: 25% of the cells have expected counts less
         than 5. Chi-Square may not be a valid test.
```

**Table 6.5** Left side: 4x2 contingency showing the SAS default sort order for a variable coded with a mixture of character and numeric data. The sort disrupts the native order of this ordinal variable. Right side: The same data as in the left panel A re-coded 1, 2, 3, 4 from lowest to highest. Re-coding aligns the native order of the variable with the program's sort instructions. Tables are rotated from the typical *y–x* orientation for formatting purposes. The statistics are not affected

The SAS System 10:15 Wednesday, September 29, 1999

TABLE OF AGE BY ND

AGE ND

| Frequency<br>Percent<br>Row Pct<br>Col Pct | 1 | 2 | Total |
|---|---|---|---|
| 60-67 | 10 | 143 | 153 |
| | 1.80 | 25.72 | 27.52 |
| | 6.54 | 93.46 | |
| | 32.26 | 27.24 | |
| 68-72 | 8 | 115 | 123 |
| | 1.44 | 20.68 | 22.12 |
| | 6.50 | 93.50 | |
| | 25.81 | 21.90 | |
| <60 | 5 | 136 | 141 |
| | 0.90 | 24.46 | 25.36 |
| | 3.55 | 96.45 | |
| | 16.13 | 25.90 | |
| >72 | 8 | 131 | 139 |
| | 1.44 | 23.56 | 25.00 |
| | 5.76 | 94.24 | |
| | 25.81 | 24.95 | |
| Total | 31 | 525 | 556 |
| | 5.58 | 94.42 | 100.00 |

The SAS System 10:15 Wednesday, September 29, 1999

TABLE OF AGEQ BY ND

AGEQ ND

| Frequency<br>Percent<br>Row Pct<br>Col Pct | 1 | 2 | Total |
|---|---|---|---|
| 1 | 5 | 136 | 141 |
| | 0.90 | 24.46 | 25.36 |
| | 3.55 | 96.45 | |
| | 16.13 | 25.90 | |
| 2 | 10 | 143 | 153 |
| | 1.80 | 25.72 | 27.52 |
| | 6.54 | 93.46 | |
| | 32.26 | 27.24 | |
| 3 | 8 | 115 | 123 |
| | 1.44 | 20.68 | 22.12 |
| | 6.50 | 93.50 | |
| | 25.81 | 21.90 | |
| 4 | 8 | 131 | 139 |
| | 1.44 | 23.56 | 25.00 |
| | 5.76 | 94.24 | |
| | 25.81 | 24.95 | |
| Total | 31 | 525 | 556 |
| | 5.58 | 94.42 | 100.00 |

The SAS System 10:15 Wednesday, September 29, 1999

STATISTICS FOR TABLE OF AGE BY ND

| Statistic | DF | Value | Prob |
|---|---|---|---|
| Chi-Square | 3 | 1.581 | 0.664 |
| Likelihood Ratio Chi-Square | 3 | 1.714 | 0.634 |
| Mantel-Haenszel Chi-Square | 1 | 0.385 | 0.535 |
| Phi Coefficient | | 0.053 | |
| Contingency Coefficient | | 0.053 | |
| Cramer's V | | 0.053 | |

Sample Size = 556

The SAS System 10:15 Wednesday, September 29, 1999

STATISTICS FOR TABLE OF AGEQ BY ND

| Statistic | DF | Value | Prob |
|---|---|---|---|
| Chi-Square | 3 | 1.581 | 0.664 |
| Likelihood Ratio Chi-Square | 3 | 1.714 | 0.634 |
| Mantel-Haenszel Chi-Square | 1 | 0.551 | 0.458 |
| Phi Coefficient | | 0.053 | |
| Contingency Coefficient | | 0.053 | |
| Cramer's V | | 0.053 | |

Sample Size = 556

In beginning the process of evaluating the effects of multiple risk factors on outcome, it can be very helpful to arrange many univariate tables into a single page of tables. This allows for visual comparisons of the relationships between variables and risk factors and gives a description of the prevalence of risk factors in the study sample. One of our favorite strategies for presenting this information is to make one large univariate table that shows many potential risk factors as they relate to the outcome. Table 6.6 is an example of our preferred format. Tables of this type, though somewhat cumbersome and time consuming to construct, contain a great deal of information that is useful to readers of study results who are interested in detailed information on the risk factors. The first things readers can determine from such tables are the prevalence and distribution of the risk factors in the population. As we have said previously, risk factor distribution is a critical factor in an investigator's evaluation of the applicability of published data to his or her own local experience. Wide diversity in risk factor distribution and prevalence between populations may lead to poor applicability of risk estimates, particularly in the multivariate setting, because of inappropriately weighted cross-population model coefficients. Comprehensive tables of this type also show univariate associations between risk factors and outcome, and statistical significance values that go with the association estimates. This allows for the examination of differences between univariate (un-adjusted) and multivariate (adjusted) estimates, and helps readers to understand confounding relationships and how risk factors relate to one another with regard to their association with the outcome. Arraying the raw data in tables also shows areas where model performance may be weak, such as associations that look important or that we would expect to be important but which are not significant because of small numbers. Only univariate statistics are shown in Table 6.6. A separate multivariate table showing the logistic regression equation needs to be examined as well to see differences between univariate and multivariate analysis results. Table 6.10 is a SAS printout that shows a logistic model with terms that are of multivariate statistical significance.

For continuous variables, and dichotomous outcomes, unpaired *t*-tests are a good univariate risk factor analysis. *t*-tests compare the means of continuous variables for two groups. So, for example, to determine

**Table 6.6** Table of univariate odds ratios by risk factor. These are unadjusted analyses. *COPD*, Chronic obstructive pulmonary disease; *TAAAII*, extent II thoracoabdominal aortic aneurysm

| Variable | No. patients | (%) | No. neurological deficit | (%) | Odds ratio* | 95% CI** | $p$*** |
|---|---|---|---|---|---|---|---|
| All patients | 556 | (100.0) | 31 | (5.6) | | | |
| Age | | | | | | | |
| 8–59 | 141 | (25.4) | 5 | (3.6) | 1.03 | 0.99–1.07 | 0.67 |
| 60–67 | 153 | (27.5) | 10 | (6.5) | | | (0.13) |
| 68–72 | 123 | (22.1) | 8 | (6.5) | | | |
| 73–88 | 139 | (25.0) | 8 | (5.8) | | | |
| Female | 196 | (35.3) | 5 | (2.6) | 0.34 | 0.13–0.89 | 0.03 |
| Male | 360 | (64.7) | 26 | (7.2) | 1 | | |
| Hypertensive | 413 | (74.3) | 23 | (5.6) | 1.00 | 0.44–2.28 | 1.00 |
| Normotensive | 143 | (25.7) | 8 | (5.6) | 1 | | |
| COPD | 178 | (32.0) | 14 | (7.9) | 1.81 | 0.87–3.77 | 0.12 |
| Otherwise | 378 | (68.0) | 17 | (4.5) | 1 | | |
| Prior | | | | | | | |
| Abdominal AA | 85 | (15.3) | 8 | (9.4) | 2.02 | 0.87–4.62 | 0.12 |
| Otherwise | 471 | (84.7) | 23 | (4.9) | 1 | | |
| Acute | | | | | | | |
| Dissection | 33 | (5.9) | 4 | (12.1) | 2.53 | 0.83–7.73 | 0.11 |
| Otherwise | 523 | (94.1) | 27 | (5.2) | 1 | | |
| Diabetes | 44 | (7.9) | 1 | (2.3) | 0.37 | 0.05–2.81 | 0.50 |
| Otherwise | 512 | (92.1) | 30 | (5.9) | 1 | | |
| Renal | | | | | | | |
| Insufficiency | 88 | (15.8) | 8 | (9.1) | 1.94 | 0.84–4.48 | 0.13 |
| Otherwise | 468 | (84.2) | 23 | (4.9) | 1 | | |
| TAAA II | 148 | (26.6) | 18 | (12.2) | 4.21 | 2.10–8.40 | 0.001 |
| Otherwise | 408 | (73.4) | 13 | (3.2) | 1 | | |

**Table 6.6** *(continued)*

| | | | | | | | |
|---|---|---|---|---|---|---|---|
| Year | | | | | | | |
| 1991 | 77 | (13.8) | 9 | (11.7) | 0.78 | 0.66–0.92 | 0.02 |
| 1992 | 61 | (11.0) | 7 | (11.5) | | | (0.004) |
| 1993 | 54 | (9.7) | 1 | (1.9) | | | |
| 1994 | 65 | (11.7) | 4 | (6.2) | | | |
| 1995 | 66 | (11.9) | 1 | (1.5) | | | |
| 1996 | 78 | (14.0) | 5 | (6.4) | | | |
| 1997 | 84 | (15.1) | 4 | (4.8) | | | |
| 1998 | 71 | (12.8) | 0 | (0.0) | | | |

*odds ratio is the common odds ratio for dichotomous data, and logistic regression odds ratio per unit change in the variable for continuous variables (age and year of surgery).
**95% CI is 95% confidence interval. It is the test-based confidence interval for dichotomous data, the maximum-likelihood confidence interval for continuous data.
***$p$ = the common $p$ value. It is chi-square probability for $2 \times 2$ tables and for $R \times C$ tables arrayed by age quartile or year. $p$ values in parentheses are $p$ values associated with logistic regression maximum likelihood estimates for continuously distributed data.

whether patients who died following coronary bypass surgery were older than patients who did not, an unpaired *t*-test could be used to compare the mean age of the two groups. A significant *p* value for the *t*-test would indicate that the average ages were different between the groups. As with all statistical tests, some requirements must be met to satisfy the test's assumptions. The continuous data need to be roughly normally distributed. A normal distribution is a standard bell-curve distribution where the mean falls in the middle and the tails are even on both sides. Figure 6.1A shows a normal distribution compared to a skewed one in Figure 6.1B. Many statistics programs will compute formal tests of distributional normality, but frequency histograms that give an eyeball sense can be useful for determining gross departure from normality as well. In cases where predictor variable data are grossly non-normal, a non-parametric test such as the Wilcoxon Rank-Sum is appropriate (10).

*t*-tests come in several varieties for specialized situations. Paired *t*-tests are for two sets of data collected from each patient (usually over time). For example, mean blood pressure before and after giving an anti-hypertensive medication would be compared by a paired *t*-test. Two or

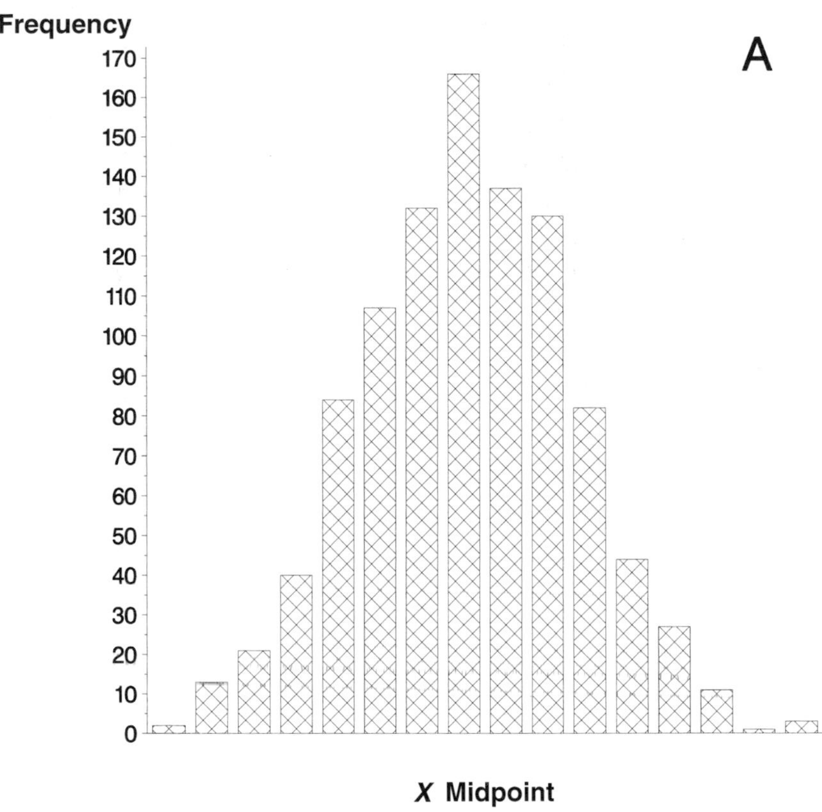


Figure 6.1 A: A normal distribution. Normal distributions have a standard bell-shaped curve and are completely described by their mean and standard deviation.

more measurements of the same variable made on one person over time are called *repeated measures*. A paired *t*-test is a very simple repeated-measures test. Risk studies do not usually involve repeated measures on individuals, and in fact repeated measures can cause problems for risk-stratification studies, particularly when the repeat is on the outcome variable. We will not go into the difficulties associated with repeated measures in risk studies, as such specialized problems are well beyond the scope of this book. Suffice it to say that repeated-measures risk factors are usually not desirable in risk studies, and repeated outcomes are to be avoided if at all possible. In circumstances where such measures are considered to be essential, repeated-measures problems *always* require the assistance of an experienced statistician.

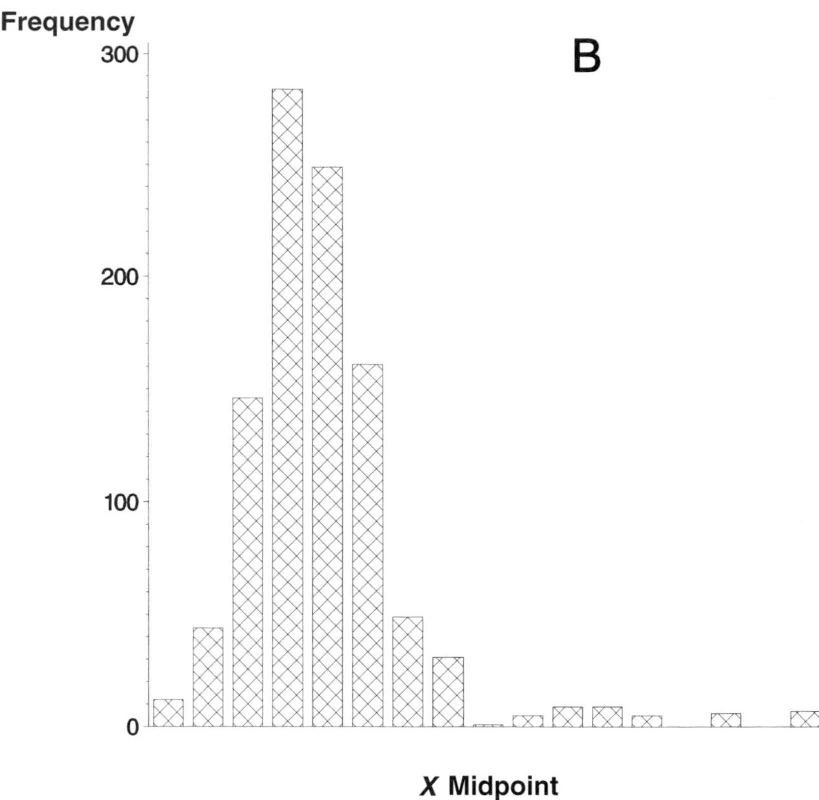


Figure 6.1 (*cont.*) B: A skewed distribution. This distribution has a normal-looking area to the left but a long right-hand tail.

Unpaired $t$-tests are appropriate for making comparisons between two groups that do not share common individuals, so an unpaired $t$-test would be used in our previous example of a comparison of ages between those who died and those who did not following coronary surgery. The unpaired test is appropriate because it is not possible for a person to be in both the dead and the surviving groups. That is, the groups represent two independent samples that share no common members. Among unpaired $t$-tests, two standard types are used. When the variation in the continuous variable is homogeneous between the two groups, an equal-variance $t$-test is used. When the variances are heterogeneous, an unequal-variance $t$-test is used. Most statistics programs will test the sample variances and report the appropriate $p$ values. SAS code for per-

**Table 6.7** SAS program that produces the univariate statistics shown in Table 6.8

```
*imported from d:\safi\thorisk2.dbf;
data risk;set thorisk2;
if preneuro ne 1;
yos=dos/365.25;
if dos ge 11323;
run;
proc sort;by ppe;run;
proc univariate plot;var age;by ppe;title;run;
proc ttest;class ppe;var age;run;
proc npar1way wilcoxon;class ppe;var age;run;
```

forming a univariate normality test, an unpaired *t*-test and a Wilcoxon Rank Sum test is shown in Table 6.7. Table 6.8 shows the program output.

In panel A of Table 6.8 we see a Univariate Procedure table for age among the patients without neurological deficit (the variable, PPE, stands for paraplegia or paraparesis = 0). When we called the Univariate Procedure in the SAS program shown toward the end of Table 6.7, we requested the "normal" and "plot" options. The "normal" option produces a *W*-test for normality, which is shown marked with an arrow. The probability value is $p < 0.0001$, which we interpret to indicate that the age distribution in the non-neurological deficit group has a highly significant departure from normality. The histogram on the page confirms this visually – we see a long-tailed distribution of ages. This is because, while the majority of patients are older people with aortic medial degenerative disease, there are a few younger people with congenital anomalies and uncommon problems such as Marfan syndrome. Seventy-five percent of the sample is over the age of 59, but the first five observations are an infant, two eight-year-olds, a 17-year-old and a 21-year-old. Observations this far from the mean are rare compared to the rest of the population, so they represent a "long tail" in the data distribution. Panel B of Table 6.8 shows the ages of patients who did not have neurological deficits. They have a much narrower age range than the

non-deficit patients, ranging from 40 to 84, and the plot shows that they are much more normal looking. The *W*-test confirms this with a *p* value of 0.3260, which would not lead us to reject the null hypothesis of normality.

In panel C of Table 6.8 we see the results of an unpaired *t*-test, which evaluates the null hypothesis that there is no difference in the average age between people with and without postoperative neurological deficit. We see that the mean age of the 525 patients without deficit is 63.89714286, and for patients with deficit it is 67.61290323. The unpaired *t*-test procedure computes both the equal-variance and the unequal-variance *t*-tests, and it also tests the sample variances to determine whether they are equal or not. In this case, we see that the hypothesis test for the equal variances assumption is $p < 0.0222$, which leads us to reject the null hypothesis that the sample variances are equal. The large differences in the histograms we saw in the Univariate Procedure output might have led us to suspect this. The *p* value for the unpaired, unequal variances *t*-test is $p < 0.0422$, which would lead us to reject the null hypothesis that the mean ages of the patients with and without a neurological deficit are the same. However, we mentioned earlier that *t*-tests require the assumption that data are fairly normally distributed, and we know that age is very non-normal in at least one group. Therefore, we should use a non-parametric test such as the Wilcoxon Rank Sum to compare the ages between groups. Non-parametric methods associate probabilities with a rank ordering of data. Rank ordering eliminates the differences in spacing between observations that would be present along the variable's normal scale, and this makes the data "distribution free". Table 6.8 panel D shows the Wilcoxon Rank Sum results. The probability of the Wilcoxon *Z*-test is $p < 0.2777$, so we do not reject the null hypothesis that age is the same between the neurological deficit and non-deficit groups. The *t*-test was fooled by the extremely non-normal distribution of the data in the non-deficit group.

Univariate tests such as these can be very helpful for evaluating the distribution of risk factors in populations and for looking at unadjusted relationships between risk factors and outcomes. Comprehensive evaluation of univariate data can help shed light on how variables influence one another when more comprehensive multivariate analyses are undertaken.

## Multivariate analysis

By far the most prevalent form of risk-stratification study performed over the last ten years has been the multivariate logistic regression study. The form of the logistic model and the rationale for its use are described in Chapter 1. Briefly, the logistic regression model is a linear model describing the relationship between a log linear combination of risk factors and the probability of an outcome. The actual running of a logistic regression model is quite easy nowadays because of the wide availability of easy-to-use software, although certain considerations in the meeting of assumptions and the selection of variables apply.

The actual programming of a logistic model involves nothing more than typing a list of variables upon which outcome probability is to be regressed. Once we have met all the requirements for data quality described previously, we proceed to the process of variable selection. Most logistic regression packages come with some form of automated model selection option. The forward selection technique allows the user to stipulate which variables will always be included in a model, but if none are specified only the model intercept is computed. Next the program calculates the statistical significance of all variables not already in the model and brings in the one with the largest chi square. It continues to bring significant variables into the model until no more significant variables are found. Once a variable is selected in, it never leaves the model. The backward elimination technique starts with a model that contains all the variable candidates specified in the program statement, and then the variables are removed one at a time starting with the least significant one. By the end of the process, all non-significant variables are eliminated. Variables are not considered again once they are eliminated. The most popular automated model selection technique is stepwise model selection, in which rotating cycles of forward and backward selection are employed to get a model that has only significant variables in it. The difference between this technique and the other two is that variables can swap in and out of stepwise models in order to maximize the number of significant variables. This is important because variables can work together in combination to cause very large reductions in the variance in the outcome prediction, so that the model may change

> **→ TIP 5**
>
> Variable selection for multivariate models is a complex process that demands great care. Over-reliance on automated variable selection techniques should be avoided.

dramatically as variables that influence one another as well as the outcome swap in and out of the model. These techniques have the virtue of being able to evaluate large numbers of possible models very quickly, but over-reliance on their use can cause numerous problems. Automated model selection techniques can be fooled by mathematical abnormalities involving high degrees of correlation or collinearity. They also consider only statistical significance in evaluating variables. Matters of biological plausibility and other considerations are beyond what automated techniques can evaluate. Appropriate selection of candidate variables in the first place will minimize problems with automated selection processes down the road.

Statistical techniques for variable selection, while they are very convenient and powerful time savers, are limited in what they can offer in terms of good model building. More important than the statistical significance of any predictor variable is its rational appropriateness. Several things need to be considered in determining the appropriateness of a multivariate model. We have already discussed the issue of pretreatment versus on- or post-treatment explanatory variables, and have indicated that pretreatment variables are usually what are desired for risk stratification. For the evaluation of pretreatment variables, one of the most important considerations is biological plausibility. It is occasionally true that peculiar correlations will appear in data – and sometimes this occurs by chance. If we were working out a model to predict the risk of mortality following coronary bypass surgery, and we found that blue eyes were a predictor of mortality, we would suspect a chance correlation. No biologically plausible mechanism by which blue eye color would increase the risk of surgical mortality has been identified, so we would in general not favor including such a variable, even if it were statistically significant, in a risk model. But blue eye color would be selected on purely statistical grounds by an automated model selection technique, so some rational control over model selection needs to be maintained by investigators. This is not to say that statistical associations may not be useful for discovery of new and previously unsuspected risk factors. Occasionally new factors are first identified by nothing more than statistical association. But in a case that is as great a stretch as blue eyes and surgical mortality, we would want to repeat the study in another group of patients before we either published the results or committed resources to trying to demonstrate a biological mechanism.

Good candidates for biologically plausible risk factors are usually things such as demographic characteristics: age, gender, body mass index, etc.; physical findings or test results related to the illness being treated – hypertension, left ventricular ejection fraction, etc. for cardiac disease; other constitutional factors such as diabetes, etc. For specialized problems, specialized risk factor variables are usually appropriate as well, and may include *previous* treatments – radiation for cancer, cardiac rehabilitation for heart disease, etc., because these often pertain to the probability of outcome following the treatment currently being planned. Variables that represent *intercurrent* treatments, even if they occur prior to the strictly defined beginning of the episode of care, are not desirable as predictors. Although these variables may account for a large amount of variance in outcome, they are too closely related to the process of care to be useful as risk-stratification variables. The purpose of risk stratification is to determine whether outcomes observed in one population differ from those that would be predicted from a standard population *on the basis of underlying severity of illness alone.* The comparisons between observed and expected outcomes are intended to adjust out differences that are attributable to severity of illness, so that residual differences can be attributed to process or quality of care. It is therefore not appropriate to use process variables to predict severity, because they are more likely to reflect the process itself rather than the underlying severity of illness in the population.

Statisticians have long held the view that the most parsimonious model that can describe a phenomenon is the most desirable one. That is, the smallest number of explanatory variables that will predict outcome accurately makes the best model. There are a number of reasons for this. Smaller models are more efficient mathematically and are easier to interpret. Fewer factors to consider leads to fewer missing data and better ascertainment.

For reasons of biological plausibility, model parsimony and avoidance of mathematical anomalies caused by high degrees of correlation and multicollinearity, variables being considered for inclusion in multivariable logistic models should be considered only because they have some likelihood of being meaningful and interpretable beyond simply being statistically significant. High capacity computers and good software can grind through a stepwise model selection using all the variables from a big database in a few seconds, so the temptation to screen huge numbers of variables is always present. We think it is bad science to take that approach, and we recommend that it should not be done even out of curiosity, because of the natural temptation to overinterpret the findings. As the computer science people like to say, "garbage in, garbage out".

## Statistical significance

We have said that statistical significance should not be the only consideration in variable selection. However, statistical significance is an important consideration when deciding whether or not to "force" a variable into a logistic model. It will occasionally be true that a variable that the investigators consider to be important will not reach statistical significance. In general, lack of statistical significance of an important-seeming variable indicates that it is not actually very important in the context of other variables. That is, other variables may confound its effects in the univariate situation and make it appear to be important when it actually is not. Multivariate modeling separates variable effects mathematically, and makes them mathematically independent. This means that influences of other variables on the effects of the variable of interest have been removed. Occasionally, however, due to low prevalence in the study sample or for other reasons, some particularly important variables that are otherwise well known to be important may not be statistically significant in a particular model. In this case, it is sometimes necessary to retain such variables in the model anyway, because their effect on other variables with regard to the outcome needs to be accounted for. Under these circumstances it is reasonable and appropriate to force a variable in; however, this should be noted and rationale given in any report that is derived from the risk-modeling project. Table 6.9 shows the final model we arrived at for predicting postoperative neurological deficit, considering all the risk factors shown in Table 6.6.

## Evaluating model prediction

We said in Chapter 1 that a variable for a logistic regression model is considered to be statistically significant when the model does a better job of matching its predictions to actual events when the variable is in the model than when the variable is out. The formal test for this is known as the likelihood ratio test, and it is the ratio of the model likelihood without a particular variable or set of variables to the model likelihood with the variable or set of variables being evaluated. The "likelihood" itself is a somewhat complicated mathematical formulation that refers to a set of regression parameters that describe the probability that a set of observed data would have occurred as a function of those parameters. Its formal specification is unnecessary for our purposes here. But the ratio of the likelihoods with and without a variable or set of variables can tell us about changes in model prediction that go with changes in variables. When the natural logarithm of the likelihood ratio is taken and multiplied by $-2$, that quantity, known as the $-2$ log likelihood, follows a known probability distribution. This probability distribution – the chi-square distribution – can be used to evaluate the statistical significance of different models with specific changes in a given set of predictor variables. Degrees of freedom for the chi-square are equal to the difference in the number of parameters between the two models being compared. The null hypothesis for the $-2$ log likelihood test is that the parameters that are different between two models being compared have coefficients equal to zero. Failure to reject the null hypothesis in a $-2$ log likelihood difference test would indicate that the parameters being evaluated are close enough to zero that they do not add significant explanatory power to the model. An example will be helpful.

In Table 6.9 we see a four-parameter logistic regression model for predicting the probability of neurological deficit following repair of thoracoabdominal aortic aneurysms. The parameters are year of surgery (YEAR), previous abdominal aortic aneurysm repair (PREVABD), extent II thoracoabdominal aortic aneurysm (TAAAII) and the model intercept (INTERCPT). The $-2$ log likelihood statistic for this model is found in the middle of the printout, and is labeled $-2$

**Table 6.9** SAS printout of multiple logistic regression analysis of risk factors for neurological deficit following aortic surgery. Predictor variables considered are those shown in Table 6.6. −2 log likelihood score for intercept only is 239.219. For the full model it is 213.056. Difference in scores is 26.163, which is chi-square distributed with three degrees of freedom (equal to the difference in number of parameters being estimated). $p$ for model −2 log likelihood is $p<0.0001$

```
                                                 10:15 Wednesday, September 29, 1999 226

                              The LOGISTIC Procedure

          Data Set: WORK.RISK
          Response Variable: PPE2
          Response Levels: 2
          Number of Observations: 556
          Link Function: Logit


                                 Response Profile

                             Ordered
                               Value     PPE2      Count

                                   1        1         31
                                   2        2        525


           Model Fitting Information and Testing Global Null Hypothesis BETA=0

                                          Intercept
                             Intercept       and
          Criterion            Only       Covariates    Chi-Square for Covariates

          AIC                241.219        221.056          .
          SC                 245.540        238.339          .
          -2 LOG L           239.219        213.056        26.163 with 3 DF (p=0.0001)
          Score                 .              .           27.253 with 3 DF (p=0.0001)


                          Analysis of Maximum Likelihood Estimates

                Parameter  Standard      Wald        Pr >      Standardized       Odds  Variable
Variable   DF    Estimate     Error  Chi-Square  Chi-Square        Estimate      Ratio    Label

INTERCPT   1      21.2346    8.8786      5.7200      0.0168               .          .  Intercept
YEAR       1      -0.2642    0.0951      7.7161      0.0055       -0.340828      0.768
PREVABD    1       1.0486    0.4551      5.3080      0.0212        0.208233      2.854  PREVABD
TAAAII     1       1.3626    0.3847     12.5452      0.0004        0.332331      3.907  TAAAII


             Association of Predicted Probabilities and Observed Responses

                       Concordant = 72.1%          Somers' D = 0.492
                       Discordant = 22.9%          Gamma     = 0.518
                       Tied       =  5.0%          Tau-a     = 0.052
                       (16275 pairs)               c         = 0.746
```

**Table 6.9** (*cont.*)

10:15 Wednesday, September 29, 1999 227

The LOGISTIC Procedure

Hosmer and Lemeshow Goodness-of-Fit Test

| | | PPE2 = 1 | | PPE2 = 2 | |
|---|---|---|---|---|---|
| Group | Total | Observed | Expected | Observed | Expected |
| 1 | 48 | 0 | 0.45 | 48 | 47.55 |
| 2 | 57 | 1 | 0.70 | 56 | 56.30 |
| 3 | 54 | 3 | 0.86 | 51 | 53.14 |
| 4 | 55 | 0 | 1.22 | 55 | 53.78 |
| 5 | 62 | 2 | 1.93 | 60 | 60.07 |
| 6 | 57 | 3 | 2.45 | 54 | 54.55 |
| 7 | 75 | 3 | 4.18 | 72 | 70.82 |
| 8 | 63 | 5 | 5.28 | 58 | 57.72 |
| 9 | 57 | 6 | 7.63 | 51 | 49.37 |
| 10 | 28 | 8 | 6.30 | 20 | 21.70 |

Goodness-of-fit Statistic = 8.753 with 8 DF (p=0.3636)

LOG L. In the column labeled "Intercept Only" we see the value 239.219, and in the column labeled "Intercept and Covariates" we see the value 213.056. The difference between these two values represents the contribution to the model's explanatory power that is made by the covariates – the predictor variables not including the intercept. That difference is 26.163. The value 26.163 follows a chi-square distribution. The intercept-only model is a one-parameter model (i.e., it contains only the model intercept), and the intercept-and-covariates model is a four-parameter model (INTERCPT, YEAR PREVABD and TAAAII). The difference in parameters between the two models is $4-1=3$. So the $-2$ log likelihood difference of 26.163 follows a chi-square distribution with three degrees of freedom – one for each parameter difference between the models. The chi-square *p* value associated with 26.163 with three degrees of freedom is $p<0.0001$. So we reject the null hypothesis that the three parameters have zero coefficients and contribute nothing to the model's explanatory power. Interpreted another way, at least one of the three parameters has a significant non-zero coefficient. This is not terribly interesting given that we already know that all the covariate model terms are significant by the Wald chi-square probabilities associated with their individual model coefficients. But we use the $-2$ log likelihood to evaluate changes in the *model performance* that are associated with the variables of interest.

Table 6.10 shows the same model as Table 6.9, with the term for PREVABD dropped out. We see that −2 LOG L in Table 6.9 is 217.756 with covariates. If we wanted to know whether the *model* (as opposed to the variable's individual statistical significance) with PREVABD in it predicted outcome better than the model without it, we could take the difference between this model's −2 log likelihood and that of the prior model with the term in. That difference would be 217.756−213.056= 4.7. Since only one parameter is different between models, 4.7 is chi-square distributed with one degree of freedom. The *p* value associated with 4.7 with one degree of freedom is $p<0.0302$, so we would reject the null hypothesis that PREVABD is unimportant. That is, we would conclude that PREVABD makes a significant improvement to the explanatory power of the model.

Only models that come from the same source data and evaluate the same variable *set* can be tested this way: −2 log likelihood comparisons between unrelated data sets would not have any meaning.

## Variable coding

Another consideration in beginning a modeling project is variable coding. We alluded to this briefly in the section above on contingency table analyses, but it is in the multivariate logistic model that this becomes a major issue. As we mentioned in previous chapters, logistic models produce regression coefficients that describe the scale of predictor variables as they relate to outcome probability. In the case of mortality following coronary bypass surgery, for example, we might find that the probability of mortality goes up by one-tenth of a percent for every year of age for ages less than 70. In the New York model the variable for years of age above 70 kicks in at age 71 and therefore adds increased risk only after age 70. So the regression coefficient for age indicates the amount of change in the predicted probability with each unit increase in age. (Remember that in a logistic model the raw predicted probability is the log odds – not the probability of the outcome. The value one-tenth of a percent is the probability converted from the odds.) For continuous

**Table 6.10** This is the model shown in Table 6.9 with the term for previous abdominal aortic aneurysm removed. −2 log likelihood for the full model is 217.756. The difference between this quantity and that of the previous model, 213.056, is 4.7. This quantity is chi-square distributed with one degree of freedom (equal to the difference in parameters being estimated between the two models). $p<0.0302$

```
                              The LOGISTIC Procedure

       Data Set: WORK.RISK
       Response Variable: PPE2
       Response Levels: 2
       Number of Observations: 556
       Link Function: Logit


                                Response Profile

                             Ordered
                               Value     PPE2      Count

                                   1        1         31
                                   2        2        525


        Model Fitting Information and Testing Global Null Hypothesis BETA=0

                                         Intercept
                          Intercept         and
      Criterion             Only         Covariates     Chi-Square for Covariates

      AIC                 241.219         223.756           .
      SC                  245.540         236.719           .
      -2 LOG L            239.219         217.756       21.463 with 2 DF (p=0.0001)
      Score                  .               .          22.500 with 2 DF (p=0.0001)


                         Analysis of Maximum Likelihood Estimates

                 Parameter  Standard      Wald        Pr >      Standardized      Odds  Variable
 Variable   DF    Estimate     Error  Chi-Square  Chi-Square      Estimate       Ratio    Label

 INTERCPT    1     18.7533    8.6046      4.7500      0.0293              .          .   Intercept
 YEAR        1     -0.2353    0.0919      6.5516      0.0105      -0.303643      0.790
 TAAAII      1      1.3203    0.3807     12.0282      0.0005       0.322003      3.745   TAAAII


          Association of Predicted Probabilities and Observed Responses
```

variables, this is a straightforward concept. But many variables are dichotomous or polychotomous (discrete values but more than two), and some way of coding these has to be worked out before they are read into a logistic model. If the database stores data for the variable "diabetes" as "yes" or "no", this will have to be re-coded for use by the model (it is difficult to multiply the term "yes"). The usual way to handle this is to code the integer value 1 for yes and 0 for no. That way, when a variable is present, it is multiplied by the regression coefficient, and when it is absent that factor is dropped out of the computations for that patient (the coefficient multiplies to zero). Polychotomous variables are somewhat different. They may be ordinal, and not meet the continuous normal distribution assumptions required for including them in the model as continuous variables. For example, thoracoabdominal aortic aneurysms are classified into five different types with regard to aneurysm extent. Type I aneurysms extend from the area just distal to the left subclavian artery to just below the diaphragm. Type II aneurysms extend from the left subclavian to below the renal arteries. Type III aneurysms extend from the sixth intercostal space to below the renal arteries. Type IV aneurysms extend from just above the diaphragm to the iliac bifurcation. Type V aneurysms extend from the sixth intercostal space to just above the renal arteries. While this variable could be coded 1 2 3 4 5 and read directly into a logistic model as though it were a continuously distributed variable, the risk associated with each value of aneurysm extent is not linear and ascending in either a continuous or an ordinal fashion. In fact, type II aneurysms carry the highest risk of postoperative spinal cord injury and mortality. The numbering system was established two decades ago, and was never intended to organize the aneurysms in order of I–V based on risk. Even if we were to re-order them according to risk, the distance between them with respect to their riskiness would not be constant. Because modeling them in a continuous distribution would lead to incorrect conclusions, we use what is known as indicator coding to identify them. With indicator coding, each aneurysm type is coded as 1 when it is present, and as 0 when it is absent. That way, the model can ascribe risk weights to each extent individually. That is, we end up with five separate indicator variables, each coded 0 or 1; one for each aneurysm extent.

We have seen that logistic regression models describe risk as the log of the odds. As we saw in Chapter 1, odds are always relative to something else. For example, the odds of dying after a coronary bypass are relative to the odds of not dying. This is particularly important where multiple indicator variables are used to describe a single ordinal classification system, as with aneurysm extent. Where we are making odds predictions conditional on the presence or absence of risk factors, the odds of an outcome in the presence of a risk factor need to be compared to the odds without the risk factor. Therefore, in logistic regression equations, it is always necessary for a reference category to exist. If we were only interested in looking at the effect of aneurysm extent on mortality in a group of surgical patients, for example, we would not get the comparisons we wanted if indicator variables for all five extents were included in the model at once. At least one would need to be left out of the model so we would have a reference for the odds predictions. If we left out type V aneurysms, for example, the odds of a postoperative death for a patient with a type II aneurysm would be as compared to a person with a type V aneurysm.

Variable coding for polychotomous classification variables is also important for −2 log likelihood testing between models. Multiple indicator variables that represent multiple levels of a single variable (aneurysm extent, quartile of age, etc.) should be moved in and out of models in blocks when making −2 log likelihood comparisons. Splitting them up is tantamount to re-coding them, because leaving some in and some out changes the reference category for the variables.

> **➔ TIP 6**
>
> Be sure to understand your software's coding conventions. Backward coding can lead to incorrect conclusions and great embarrassment.

It is often necessary to make a few minor adjustments to the standard coding conventions to accommodate software idiosyncrasies and to meet certain assumptions. Some statistics programs require different variable coding for different situations. In the case of SAS, the coding for tables is different from that for logistic regression. These requirements affect both univariate and multivariate analyses. For example, in the SAS version of the aortic dissection univariate analysis that we went through earlier (Table 6.4), note that presence of a condition (either dissection or paraplegia) is denoted by a 1, which is conventional. But *absence* of a condition, instead of using the conventional 0 coding, is coded as a 2. This is because SAS sorts variable values in ascending order, so that the tables are arrayed with the smallest variable values first, and with the larger values following in order. If we had used the conventional 0,1 coding, absent risk factor and absent outcome would be the first cells in the rows and columns because of the sort order. That would not matter for the significance tests, which look only at association between rows and columns, but the odds ratio would be inverted. In Table 6.1, the odds ratio was (4/29)/(27/496) = 2.53. If the table were arrayed the other way, the odds ratio would be (27/496)/(4/29) = 0.395. So if we forgot to change the coding for dissection and neurological deficit from 1,0 to 1,2 before doing this analysis, we could be fooled into thinking that the odds ratio was 0.395 instead of 2.53, and that dissection was actually protective against neurological deficit. The main thing to keep in mind when coding tables is to keep the concordant (risk = yes outcome = yes, risk = no outcome = no) table cells on the main diagonal. The main diagonal is the one that goes from upper left to lower right.

Coding order is important for logistic models as well, but for a different reason. As we can easily see, 1,2 coding for logistic *predictor* (i.e., risk factor) variables would not give the results we were after, because using 2 to denote absence of a risk factor would cause the regression coefficient to be multiplied by 2 instead of 0 when the risk factor was absent. 0,1 coding must be maintained for indicator *predictor* variables in logistic models. However SAS in particular codes the *outcome* variable for a logistic equation 1,2, because it takes the outcome variable values in sorted order and assumes that the first value is outcome = yes. This is tremendously important when using SAS, because if the outcome variable is coded 1,0 the risk factor estimates will be inverted, as we saw in the contingency table example. If the factors are inverted, something that is actually harmful will look protective. Coding rules for software programs may vary procedure by procedure, and it is essential that the investigator be clear about what the coding means before beginning model construction.

One final detail with regard to variable coding is as follows. Missing data should not be coded as zero. A missing data point is not the same as one in which the risk factor is absent, and the computer reads a risk factor coded as zero as the patient not having the risk factor. Improper coding of missing data is a problem for all types of data, whether discrete or continuous. A missing value for ejection fraction, for example, is not the same as an ejection fraction of zero, which would not be a physiologically survivable situation. If we don't know whether a person has had a myocardial infarction in the past six months, that does not mean that the person has not had one. If in fact the person has had an infarct and we code it as zero or "no", then we have made a classification error with regard to this person's risk factors. Very many of these misclassifications in a study sample will bias the results in ways that we have described previously. Always denote missing data with a period or a blank.

## Fit testing

Several methods for testing the fit of logistic regression models have been described, but the one that is most widely used is the Hosmer–Lemeshow test (12). We talked in Chapter 1 about statistical significance testing for logistic models, and about how part of the process involved comparing the classification accuracy of the model with a particular variable included in the model to the classification accuracy of the model with the variable out. The Hosmer–Lemeshow test extends this concept by computing a test of classification accuracy across a wide range of model prediction values, and then breaking the classification down into zones to see where classification is best and where it is worst. Hosmer–Lemeshow breaks the range of model prediction into roughly ten categories or probability zones, and then computes a significance test to see how well predicted probabilities go with the events for each level of predicted probability. If the significance test has a low $p$ value (i.e., less that 0.05), the null hypothesis that the actual events go with the predictions across the range of prediction is rejected, and the model is said to lack proper fit. To get the Hosmer–Lemeshow statistic, the lack of fit option is specified in the logistic regression procedure (Table 6.11 shows the SAS code). Table 6.12 shows the output for the lack of fit test. Below the title "Hosmer and Lemeshow Goodness-of-Fit Test" we see two major headings, PPE2 = 1 and PPE2 = 2. The variable PPE is paraplegia or paraparesis immediately following a thoracoabdominal aortic aneurysm repair operation. PPE2 is the 1,0 (yes, no) PPE variable re-coded as 1,2 for use as a SAS logistic *outcome* variable. Below the PPE2 titles we see columns entitled Group, Total, and two sets of Observed and Expected values; one set for PPE2 = 1 (paraplegia or paraparesis present), and one set for PPE2 = 2 (paraplegia or paraparesis not present). The group variable indicates that the

**Table 6.11** SAS code that produces the logistic regression model shown in Table 6.12 with the Hosmer–Lemeshow lack-of-fit test requested

```
*imported from d:\safi\thorisk2.dbf;
data risk;set thorisk2;
format dos yymmdd2.;
format age 2.;
format ppe 3.1;
if dos ge 11323 and dos le 11687 then year=91;
if dos ge 11688 and dos le 12053 then year=92;
if dos ge 12054 and dos le 12418 then year=93;
if dos ge 12419 and dos le 12783 then year=94;
if dos ge 12784 and dos le 13148 then year=95;
if dos ge 13149 and dos le 13514 then year=96;
if dos ge 13515 and dos le 13879 then year=97;
if dos ge 13880 and dos le 14244 then year=98;
if age gt 0 and age le 59 then ageq=1;
if age ge 60 and age le 67 then ageq=2;
if age ge 68 and age le 72 then ageq=3;
if age ge 73 then ageq=4;
if edeath=1 then edeath2=1;else edeath2=2;
if ppe=1 then ppe2=1;else ppe2=2;
if ppl=1 then ppl2=1;else ppl2=2;
if taaaii=1 then taaaii2=1;
if taaaii=0 then taaaii2=2;
if taaaiii=1 then taaaiii2=1;
if taaaiii=0 then taaaiii2=2;
if copd=1 then copd2=1;
if copd=0 then copd2=2;
if acuted=1 then acute2=1;
if acuted=0 then acute2=2;
if diabetes=1 then diab2=1;
if diabetes=0 then diab2=2;
if htn=1 then htn2=1;
if htn=0 then htn2=2;
if prevabd=1 then prevabd2=1;
if prevabd=0 then prevabd2=2;
if rup=1 then rup2=1;
if rup=0 then rup2=2;
if renins=1 then renins2=1;
if renins=0 then renins2=2;
if prevtaaa=1 then prevtaa2=1;
if prevtaaa=0 then prevtaa2=2;
if atype='DESC' then desc=1;else desc=0;
if sex='F' or sex='f' then female=1;else female=0;
if female=1 then fem2=1;
if female=0 then fem2=2;
if preneuro ne 1;
yos=dos/365.25;
if dos ge 11323;
run;
proc logistic;model ppe2=year prevabd taaaii / lackfit;
run;
```

**Table 6.12** This is the logistic regression model shown in Table 6.9. The probability range is separated into ten zones and observed events and those expected by the model are compared. No significant departure from good fit is detected. $p = 0.3636$

```
                                        10:15 Wednesday, September 29, 1999

                          The LOGISTIC Procedure

        Data Set: WORK.RISK
        Response Variable: PPE2
        Response Levels: 2
        Number of Observations: 556
        Link Function: Logit

                             Response Profile

                          Ordered
                            Value     PPE2      Count

                                1        1         31
                                2        2        525

      Model Fitting Information and Testing Global Null Hypothesis BETA=0

                                   Intercept
                      Intercept       and
        Criterion       Only      Covariates   Chi-Square for Covariates

        AIC            241.219       221.056          .
        SC             245.540       238.339          .
        -2 LOG L       239.219       213.056       26.163 with 3 DF (p=0.0001)
        Score             .             .          27.253 with 3 DF (p=0.0001)

                     Analysis of Maximum Likelihood Estimates

                Parameter  Standard      Wald        Pr >    Standardized      Odds  Variable
Variable   DF    Estimate     Error  Chi-Square  Chi-Square      Estimate     Ratio   Label

INTERCPT    1     21.2346    8.8786      5.7200      0.0168             .         .  Intercept
YEAR        1     -0.2642    0.0951      7.7161      0.0055     -0.340828     0.768
PREVABD     1      1.0486    0.4551      5.3080      0.0212      0.208233     2.854  PREVABD
TAAAII      1      1.3626    0.3847     12.5452      0.0004      0.332331     3.907  TAAAII

          Association of Predicted Probabilities and Observed Responses

                     Concordant = 72.1%          Somers' D = 0.492
                     Discordant = 22.9%          Gamma     = 0.518
                     Tied       =  5.0%          Tau-a     = 0.052
                     (16275 pairs)               c         = 0.746

                                   10:15 Wednesday, September 29, 1999

               The LOGISTIC Procedure

        Hosmer and Lemeshow Goodness-of-Fit Test

                        PPE2 = 1                  PPE2 = 2
                  --------------------      --------------------
Group      Total  Observed    Expected      Observed    Expected

  1          48          0        0.45            48       47.55
  2          57          1        0.70            56       56.30
  3          54          3        0.86            51       53.14
  4          55          0        1.22            55       53.78
  5          62          2        1.93            60       60.07
  6          57          3        2.45            54       54.55
  7          75          3        4.18            72       70.82
  8          63          5        5.28            58       57.72
  9          57          6        7.63            51       49.37
 10          28          8        6.30            20       21.70

     Goodness-of-fit Statistic = 8.753 with 8 DF (p=0.3636)
```

Hosmer–Lemeshow test stratified the sample into ten risk categories or probability zones for comparison of observed to expected events. These occur in ascending order of paraplegia/paraparesis risk, and they are classified by the risk expectations produced by a logistic regression model that we will examine in more detail in the section on interpretation at the end of the chapter. The column labeled total is the number of patients in each risk stratum. Observed under PPE2 = 1 is the number of paraplegias/parapareses observed in that particular risk stratum. Expected is the number of events expected by the model based on risk factors. For the Observed and Expected columns under PPE2 = 2 are the number of non-events observed (i.e., patients who recovered from surgery successfully without paraplegia or paraparesis), and the number of non-events expected. We see in the first zone of the observed column for PPE2 = 1 that 0 events were observed in that risk stratum, while 0.45 were expected based on the model. As we move further down the list both the observed and the expected numbers of events go up. In the third stratum, three events are observed where 0.86 would have been expected, but other than that the observed and expected are very close. We see that the $p$ value shown in parentheses at the bottom confirms this: $p = 0.3636$, which is nowhere near significant. So we conclude that the model does not demonstrate a significant departure from a good fit. Fit testing should always be done when a modeling project is getting on toward its final stages. This helps to identify weak areas of model performance and to assist in determining the overall accuracy of model predictions across the range of the dependent variable.

## Plotting

Plotting data is another good way to evaluate the accuracy of a model and to understand what it is telling us about the relationship between risk factors and outcome. Plotting probability data is a somewhat different process from plotting more commonly shown linear regression data. In linear models, explanatory variables are used to predict the mean of a normal-continuous response variable over a range of explanatory variable values. The values of the response variable are actual observations that can be plotted on a scatter diagram. Figure 6.2 shows a scatter plot with two continuous variables. The regression function (described by the

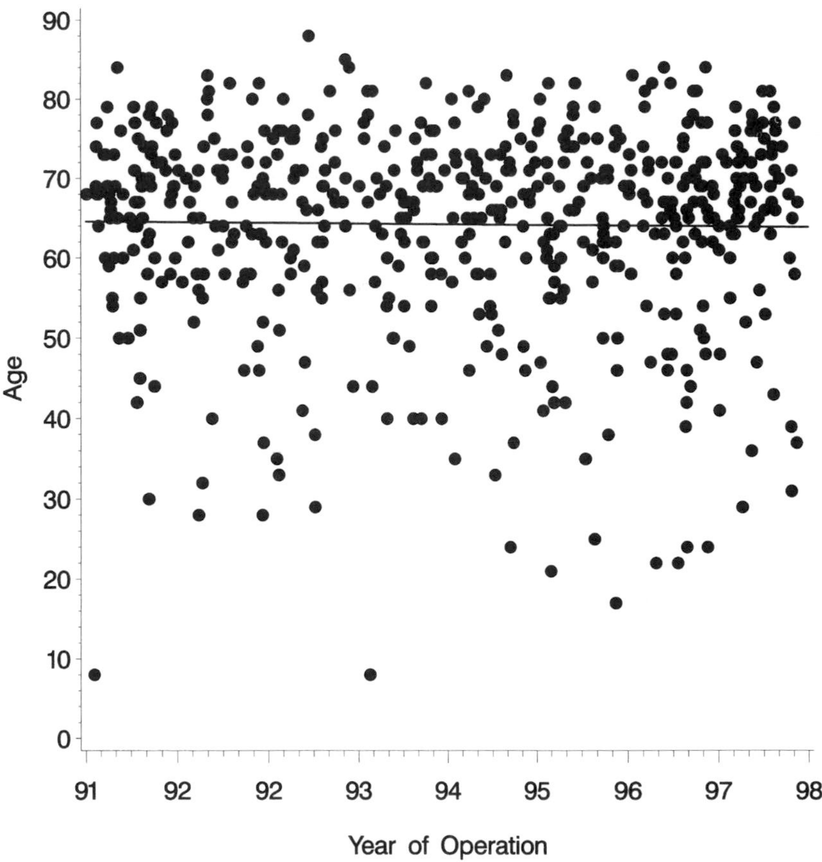


Figure 6.2 Traditional scatter plot of two continuously distributed variables, in this case age and year of operation. Data points can fall anywhere along either axis. Data points are plotted daily with the *x*-axis marked every 365 days; hence, 1992 is marked twice as it was a leap year

regression line) for a linear regression model is the mean of the response variable spread across the range of the predictor variable.

The *actual* response variable data for a logistic regression model are different from linear model response data, because they do not fall over a continuum as continuous data do. That is, the *actual* data (not the modeled log odds) for a logistic regression response variable can only take one of two values – present or absent (1 or 2 in SAS coding). If we were to plot the actual values of the logistic model response variable, the values on the response axis could only take on the values 0 for outcome

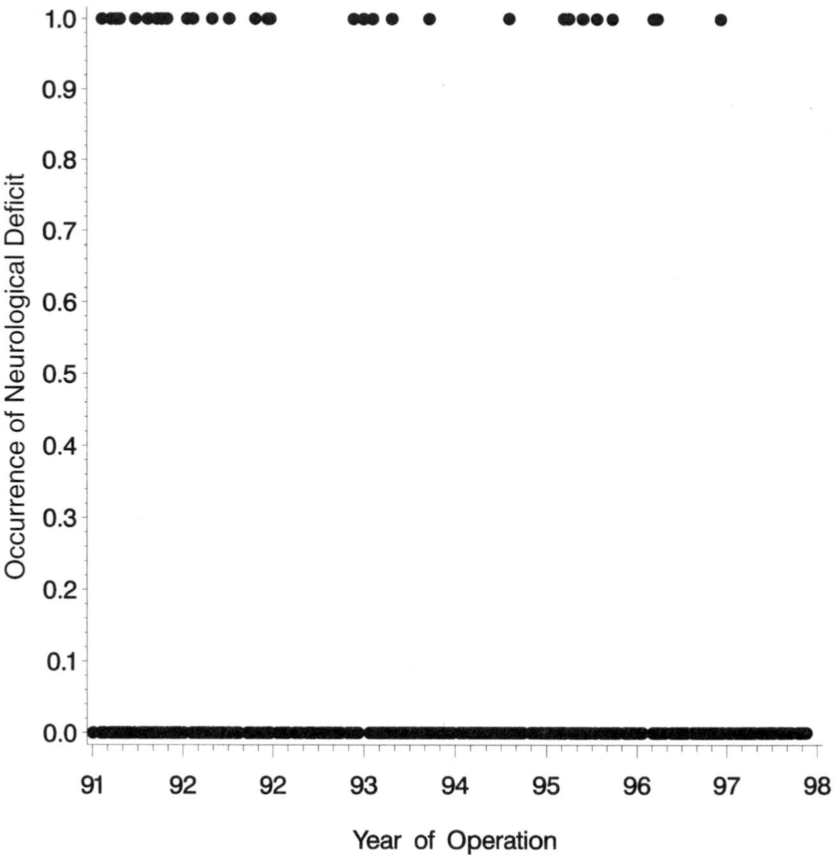


Figure 6.3 Plot of neurological deficit occurrence versus non-occurrence plotted against year of operation. Neurological deficit can only take on two values, zero (no) and 1 (yes). This type of plot tells us very little about the occurrence of neurological deficit over time.

absent and 1 for outcome present. This would cause them to line up in two rows against the range of the predictor variable, and it would be quite difficult to determine the relationship between the predictor variable and the probability of the dichotomous response. Figure 6.3 shows dichotomous outcome data, postoperative neurological deficit or not, plotted against year of surgery. This is what we might call a "hindsight" plot. Patients who actually had a neurological deficit following surgery had a 100 percent chance of having one, while patients who did not have one had a zero percent chance, in hindsight. Unfortunately, these hindsight probabilities are not terribly instructive for predicting events in the future, because predictive probabilities vary more than hindsight ones. With the outcomes all lined up along the top and the bottom of the plot, it is also difficult to tell how the events aggregate relative to the non-events. There are too many overlapping points to be able to see how they lie.

What we would prefer to have rather than hindsight probabilities stacked on top of each other is some sort of a probability function that describes predicted probability in a way that we can interpret it. The logistic model allows us to calculate log odds based on predictor variables and to convert those values to probabilities. Figure 6.4 shows the data from the plot in Figure 6.3 with the logistic probability prediction line superimposed. We see that in 1991 the probability of a postoperative neurological deficit is around 11 percent, but by 1998 it had dropped to around two percent. This would be very hard to ascertain from the raw plot by itself. Plotting the response function as a probability describes the relationship between the risk factor values and the predicted probability of an event in a way simply arraying the data does not.

In the univariate logistic regression situation, plotting data can also be very useful for checking the accuracy of logistic models. Data can be arrayed into discrete units of the continuous variable (e.g., year of operation, quartile of age, etc.), risk can be computed for each of the discrete units, and then the continuous risk estimate and the discrete risk can be plotted alongside one another. Figure 6.5 shows a continuous probability function over year of operation plotted alongside data compartmentalized into discrete form by year.

Probability is plotted by multiplying a range of predictor variable values through the model coefficients, and then converting the resulting odds to probabilities. Table 6.13 shows the SAS code for producing the probability plots shown in Figures 6.2–6.4. Appendix 3 gives a line-by-line explanation of the program.

## Interpretation

Logistic models are interpreted first according to numerous criteria that we have already mentioned. Biological plausibility, model fit, explanatory power of the model based on statistical criteria, and utility of the

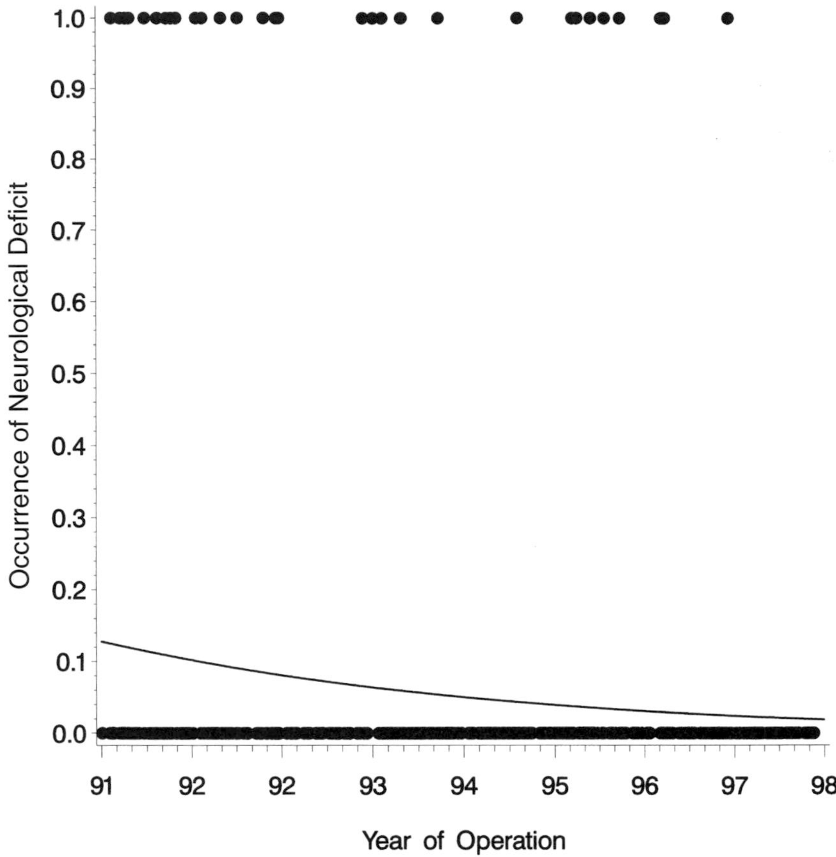


Figure 6.4 The same plot as Figure 6.3 with a logistic-regression-predicted probability line superimposed. The probability estimate shows us that risk was highest initially and comes down over time. The logistic regression curve makes the unintelligible data in Figure 6.3 easy to interpret.

model in classifying events are some of these. We noted in Chapter 1 that multiple logistic regression is a technique by which we can make adjustments for dependencies, or non-independence, between risk factor variables and the outcome. By using mathematics to sort out the dependencies, we can evaluate the amount of confounding or overlap between predictor variables as these relate to the outcome, by comparing univariate associations between risk factors and outcomes to multivariate associations. We saw earlier in this chapter how odds ratios are computed from contingency table data. Logistic regression analysis can

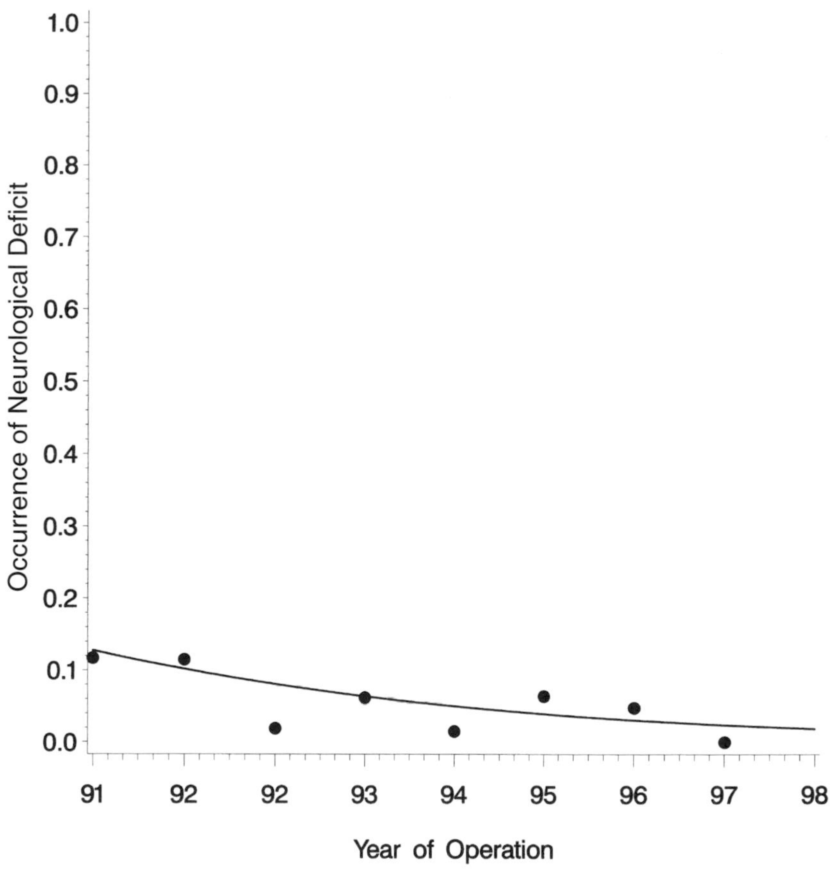


Figure 6.5 Dots represent data shown in Figures 6.3 and 6.4 aggregated by year and expressed as proportions per year. The same logistic curve as in Figure 6.4 is shown. The curve does a very good job of summarizing the probability (i.e., the relative frequency or proportion) of neurological deficit over time, and therefore is an accurate reflection of the actual population experience.

be used to compute adjusted multivariate odds ratios for several risk factors simultaneously.

When we applied published logistic formulas that had been derived from external populations in Chapter 4, we did not worry about the interpretation of the individual regression coefficients beyond summing them up and solving the equations for summary odds. We did not need to worry about odds *ratios* for the individual variables – those were

**Table 6.13** SAS code for producing Figures 6.2–6.4. A line-by-line explanation of this program is shown in Appendix 3

```
*imported from d:\safi\thorisk2.dbf;
data risk;set thorisk2;
format dos yymmdd2.;
format age 2.;
format ppe 3.1;
if dos ge 11323 and dos le 11687 then year=91;
if dos ge 11688 and dos le 12053 then year=92;
if dos ge 12054 and dos le 12418 then year=93;
if dos ge 12419 and dos le 12783 then year=94;
if dos ge 12784 and dos le 13148 then year=95;
if dos ge 13149 and dos le 13514 then year=96;
if dos ge 13515 and dos le 13879 then year=97;
if dos ge 13880 and dos le 14244 then year=98;
if age gt 0 and age le 59 then ageq=1;
if age ge 60 and age le 67 then ageq=2;
if age ge 68 and age le 72 then ageq=3;
if age ge 73 then ageq=4;
if edeath=1 then edeath2=1;else edeath2=2;
if ppe=1 then ppe2=1;else ppe2=2;
if ppl=1 then ppl2=1;else ppl2=2;
if taaaii=1 then taaaii2=1;
if taaaii=0 then taaaii2=2;
if taaaiii=1 then taaaiii2=1;
if taaaiii=0 then taaaiii2=2;
if copd=1 then copd2=1;
if copd=0 then copd2=2;
if acuted=1 then acute2=1;
if acuted=0 then acute2=2;
if diabetes=1 then diab2=1;
if diabetes=0 then diab2=2;
if htn=1 then htn2=1;
if htn=0 then htn2=2;
if prevabd=1 then prevabd2=1;
if prevabd=0 then prevabd2=2;
if rup=1 then rup2=1;
if rup=0 then rup2=2;
if renins=1 then renins2=1;
if renins=0 then renins2=2;
if prevtaaa=1 then prevtaa2=1;
if prevtaaa=0 then prevtaa2=2;
if atype='DESC' then desc=1;else desc=0;
if sex='F' or sex='f' then female=1;else female=0;
if female=1 then fem2=1;
if female=0 then fem2=2;
if preneuro ne 1;
run;
proc sort;by dos;run;
data risk2;
do dos=11323 to 14244 by 1;
o=exp(6.0061+(dos*-0.0007));
p=o/(1+o);
output;
end;
run;
proc sort;by dos;run;
data both;merge risk risk2;by dos;run;
goptions device=winprtg htext=1 ftext=swiss;
axis1 length=15 cm label=(a=90 r=0);
axis2 length=15 cm order=(11323 to 14244 by 365);
symbol v=dot i=rl;
proc gplot data=risk;plot age*dos / vaxis=axis1 haxis=axis2;
label age='Age';
label dos='Year of Operation';
run;
goptions device=winprtg htext=1 ftext=swiss;
axis1 length=15 cm label=(a=90 r=0) order=(0 to 1 by 0.1);
axis2 length=15 cm order=(11323 to 14244 by 365);
symbol v=dot i=none;
proc gplot data=risk;plot ppe*dos / vaxis=axis1 haxis=axis2;
label ppe='Occurrence of Neurologic Deficit';
label dos='Year of Operation';
run;
goptions device=winprtc htext=1 ftext=swiss;
axis1 length=15 cm label=(a=90 r=0) order=(0 to 1 by 0.1);
axis2 length=15 cm order=(11323 to 14244 by 365);
symbol2 v=dot i=none c=black;
symbol1 v=none i=join w=10 c=black;
proc gplot data=both;plot (p ppe)*dos / overlay vaxis=axis1 haxis=axis2;
label p='Probability of Neurologic Deficit';
label dos='Year of Operation';
run;
proc print;run;
```

established by the original population to which the model was fitted – and would not ordinarily be of interest in the process of risk stratification using outside equations. The odds ratios would be fixed to the source population, and we would only be looking to see whether our outcomes matched those expected by the published fixed-coefficient model we were using. The authors of the published study would have dealt with variable interactions and odds ratio/magnitude of association issues in the process of analyzing their own data.

But in fitting our own logistic regression model to local data, we are extremely interested in how odds associated with predictors in our own study sample are affected by inclusion and exclusion of multiple predictor variables, because these issues are germane to variable selection and construction of the final model. Recommendations vary among the experts for the way variables evaluated in univariate analysis are brought into multivariate models. Some authors recommend considering all univariate associations with $p$ values less than 0.10 in multivariate models. This is an arbitrary statistical criterion, and our preference is not to make decisions based on statistical criteria alone. We prefer to evaluate all variables that have a reasonable, biologically plausible likelihood of contributing explanatory variance reduction to the outcome of interest. We usually make a run at stepwise modeling then go back with forward selection, forcing in any variables we consider it necessary to account for. Once we have evaluated all the variables that are either statistically significant in automated selection or that we have forced in based on *a priori* criteria, we put the model together one variable at a time manually, until we are satisfied that we understand how variables relate to one another and influence one another with regard to the outcome. Being thus satisfied, we look at fit, at probability plots and at the multivariate odds ratios described by each variable's regression coefficient.

We have said in several places in this book that the endproduct of a logistic regression model is the log odds, which can be converted to odds and then to probability. Each regression coefficient can also be evaluated by itself as an adjusted odds ratio. Simply taking the exponent of any first-order (i.e., not including interaction terms or other non-linear terms) logistic regression coefficient gives an estimate of the adjusted odds ratio for that variable. For example, to get the adjusted odds ratio for previous abdominal aortic aneurysm repair, we would simply take the exponent of that term's regression coefficient, exp(1.0486) = 2.854. We call it an adjusted odds ratio because it is the variable's odds ratio that is adjusted for the effects of the other variables by multidimensional mathematics. If we construct a large table of univariate results as we showed in Table 6.6, we can compare the multivariate results to the univariate results to see how much overlap exists between the explanatory variables with respect to the outcome. This is a major issue in interpreting the results of logistic regression models, and the results of studies based on local data generally.

Recall that Table 6.9 shows a logistic regression analysis of the same data that were subjected to univariate analysis in Table 6.6. We see that the final model contains the variables year of surgery (YEAR), history of a previous abdominal aortic aneurysm repair (PREVABD), and Crawford aneurysm extent II (TAAAII). All of these variables are statistically significant. We saw in the section above on goodness-of-fit that the model fits well. This is the same model that produced the Hosmer–Lemeshow results shown in Table 6.12. Since we have a model that we are satisfied with in terms of all the criteria we have described at length previously, we can compare the estimated univariate odds ratios with the multivariate ones. Table 6.14 simplifies this comparison. On the left we see the univariate odds ratios and $p$ values, on the right, the multivariate values. The first pattern we notice is that the multivariate $p$ values tend to be lower than the univariate $p$ values. This can be somewhat difficult to interpret, because it can mean that the model is over-fitted to the data, but SAS will usually issue a warning when combinations of variables work together to cause over-fit instability in the model, or a "quasi-complete separation" in the response. In this particular case, it is more likely that the variables taken in combination explain more of the variance in outcome than they do taken separately, so that uncertainty is reduced and alpha error probabilities are reduced as a consequence. The odds ratios are also adjusted for the effects on one another. In the example shown in the table, the univariate and multivariate odds ratio estimates are quite close. The effect of extent II aneurysm is reduced somewhat in the multivariate scenario, but this is because year of surgery is included in the model. As we mentioned earlier, operative techniques

**Table 6.14** Side-by-side comparison of univariate and multivariate test results of significant predictors of neurological deficit. The results are pretty close, although the magnitude of the effect of type-II aneurysm is somewhat reduced in the multivariate model. This is because the risk associated with type-II aneurysm comes down over time, and the variable that captures the effect of year accounts for some of the variance

| | Univariate estimate | | Multivariate estimate | |
|---|---|---|---|---|
| Variable | Odds ratio | *p* | Odds ratio | *p* |
| Year of surgery | 0.78 | 0.004 | 0.77 | 0.006 |
| Previous abdominal aneurysm surgery | 2.02 | 0.12 | 2.86 | 0.03 |
| Extent II Aneurysm | 4.21 | 0.001 | 3.91 | 0.0004 |

have improved over time, and this has helped to mitigate the risk associated with extent II aneurysms. This effect is apparent in the estimates that reflect process of care even without the inclusion of process of care variables. The many stages of analysis can tell us many things about our data and about the way multiple factors work together to influence the probability of outcome.

## Conclusion

In this chapter we have described the process of constructing a *de novo* risk-stratification study from local data, that could be used by other investigators as a standardization study. Risk-stratification studies are typically observational in design, and they are necessarily prospective in directionality because the relationship (i.e., the relative frequency) between events and non-events must be maintained for prediction. Case–control studies can be useful for identifying risk factors that can be used in prospective studies later on, but case–control designs do not provide the data on incidence that are necessary for modeling risk. Because other investigators at other institutions may wish to use the results of this type of study in their own standardization projects, careful attention must be paid to the details of case ascertainment, competing risks and the like. Details of techniques for case ascertainment, as well as case and variable definition, must be included in reports intended for publication or for any outside use. Good documentation of these things is essential for the ability of others to apply the estimates to their own local data. Comprehensive univariate and multivariate examinations of the data should be undertaken, and tables that describe the prevalence of the risk factors and the outcome in the source population should be constructed. Models should be constructed by a combination of statistical significance testing and rational planning, with particular attention to the biological plausibility and the conceptual appropriateness of variables that will ultimately be used to make inferences about the quality and process of care. Regression diagnostics such as fit testing and plots are also appropriate measures for evaluating the quality of multivariate statistical models. Ultimately, the goal of a *de novo* risk modeling project should be to produce a model that makes sense in the context in which it will be used, and that will assist others working in the field with the interpretation and modification of their own processes of care.

## REFERENCES

1 Miller CC, III, Safi HJ, Winnerkvist A, Baldwin JC. Actual vs. actuarial analysis for cardiac valve complications: the problem of competing risks. *Curr Opin Cardiol* 1999; **14**: 79–83.

2 Safi HJ, Miller CC, III, Azizzadeh A, Iliopoulos DC. Observations on delayed neurologic deficit after thoracoabdominal aortic aneurysm repair. *J Vasc Surg* 1997; **26**: 616–22.

3 Safi HJ, Campbell MP, Miller CC, III, Iliopoulos DC, Khoynezhad AK, Letsou GV, Asimacopoulos PJ. Cerebral spinal fluid drainage and distal aortic perfusion decrease the incidence of neurologic deficit: the results of 343 descending and thoracoabdominal aortic aneurysm repairs. *Eur J Vasc Endovasc Surg* 1997; **14**: 118–24.

4 Safi HJ, Campbell MP, Ferreira ML, Azizzadeh A, Miller CC, III. Spinal cord protection in descending thoracic and thoracoabdominal aortic aneurysm repair. *Semin Thorac Cardiovasc Surg* 1998; **10**: 41–4.

5 Safi HJ, Miller CC, III, Carr C, Iliopoulos DC, Dorsay DA Baldwin JC. Importance of intercostal artery reattachment during thoracoabdominal aortic aneurysm repair. *J Vasc Surg* 1998; **27**: 58–68.

6 Safi HJ, Miller CC, III, Reardon MJ, Iliopoulos DC, Letsou GV, Espada R, Baldwin JC. Operation for acute and chronic aortic dissection: recent outcome with regard to neurologic deficit and early death. *Ann Thorac Surg* 1998; **66**: 402–11.

7 Safi HJ, Vinnerkvist A, Miller CC, III, Iliopoulos DC, Reardon MJ, Espada R, Baldwin JC. Effect of extended cross-clamp time during thoracoabdominal aortic aneurysm repair. *Ann Thorac Surg* 1998; **66**: 1204–9.

8 Safi HJ, Miller CC, III. Spinal cord protection in descending thoracic and thoracoabdominal aortic repair. *Ann Thorac Surg* 1999; **67**: 1937–9.

9 Safi HJ, Subramaniam MH, Miller CC, III, Coogan SM, Iliopoulos DC, Vinnerkvist A, LeBlevec D, Bahnini A. Progress in the management of type I thoracoabdominal and descending aortic aneurysms. *Ann Vasc Surg* 1999; **13**: 457–62.

10 Rosner B. *Fundamentals of Biostatistics*, third edition. PWS Kent, Boston, 1990.

11 Svensson LG, Crawford ES, Hess KR, Coselli JS, Safi HJ. Experience with 1509 patients undergoing thoracoabdominal aortic operations. *J Vasc Surg* 1993; **17**: 357–68.

12 Hosmer DW, Lemeshow S. *Applied Logistic Regression*. John Wiley & Sons, New York, 1989.

# Appendix 1 SAS code to produce the print in Table 4.5

```
1  data ch4;
2  infile 'd:\bookstat\ch4dat.txt' missover lrecl=265;
3  informat doadmit datesurg datedis mmddyy8.;
4  format doadmit datesurg datedis mmddyy8.;
5  input counter 1-10 encounte 12-26 lname$ 28-62 fname$ 64-98 surgeon$ 100-134
6   drg 136-141 doadmit age 152-154 height 156-161 weight 163-168 female 170
7   smoke 172 packs 174-179 yrs 181-186 lmain 188 uangina 190 sangina 192
8   ptcaemer 194 ivnitr 196 ivinotr 198 ef 200-205 novessel 207 venaneu 209
9   mi7d 211 mi24h 213 mi3wk 215 migt3wk 217 balpump 219 chf 221 structur 223
10  renfail 225 shock 227 htn 229 diabetes 231 copd 233 dialysis 235 CVD 237
11  valvdis 239 prevsurg 241 datesurg datedis death 261 priority 263;
12 htm=(height*2.54)/100;
13 wtk=weight/2.2;
14 bmi=wtk/(htm**2);
15 if bmi ge 39 then mobesity=1;else mobesity=0;
16 pyears=packs*yrs;
17 if smoke=1 and packs=0 then pyears=.;
18 if ef=0 then ef=.;
19 if ef gt  0 and ef lt 20 then eflt20=1;else eflt20=0;
20 if ef ge 20 and ef lt 30 then ef2029=1;else ef2029=0;
21 if ef ge 30 and ef lt 40 then ef3039=1;else ef3039=0;
22 if ef=. then efmiss=1;else efmiss=0;
23 if mi7d=1 or mi24h=1 then recentmi=1;else recentmi=0;
24 if prevsurg gt 0 then prevop=1;else prevop=0;
25 if age gt 70 then m70=age-70;
26 if age le 70 then m70=0;
27 if structur=1 or renfail=1 or shock=1 then disast=1;else disast=0;
28 mortodds=exp(-6.9605+(age*0.0346)+(m70*0.0439)+(female*0.4154)+
29  (lmain*0.3612)+(uangina*0.3533)+(eflt20*1.4008)+(ef2029*0.7920)+
30  (ef3039*0.4881)+(efmiss*0.4810)+(recentmi*0.5253)+(balpump*0.3284)+
31  (chf*0.5684)+(disast*1.3814)+(diabetes*0.4029)+(mobesity*0.3961)+
32  (copd*0.3063)+(dialysis*1.0281)+(prevop*1.3174));
33 probmort=mortodds/(1+mortodds);
34 pctmort=probmort*100;
35 run;
36 proc print;var age m70 female lmain uangina eflt20 ef2029 ef3039 efmiss recentmi
37  balpump chf disast diabetes mobesity copd dialysis prevop mortodds probmort pctmort;
38 run;
```

*Line 1* names the data set.

*Line 2* reads in the data from an ASCII text file called ch4dat.txt that is located on the d: drive in a folder called bookstat. The missover command instructs the SAS pointer that keeps track of observations to skip missing data points rather than to continue on to the next column or line looking for them. The lrecl command specifies the length of the logical record, or the number of characters and spaces in a single row of data in the file.

*Line 3* specifies the format that date variables are in when they are read in, and *line 4* tells SAS how to format the date variables for printing.

*Line 5* begins the input statement, which tells SAS the variable names, variable types and gives physical locations for the data in the infile. "Counter" is the first variable, and is located between spaces 1 and 10 in the input file. All variables are assumed to be numeric unless otherwise specified. The variable lname$ is last name, which is character. Character variables are denoted with a $.

*Line 12* converts height in inches to meters.

*Line 13* converts weight in pounds to kilograms.

*Line 14* calculates body mass index (BMI).

*Line 15* sets the value of the variable for morbid obesity to one if BMI is 39 or above, to zero otherwise.

*Line 16* calculates pack-years of smoking.

*Line 17* sets the value of pack-years to missing if current smoking is indicated but the number of packs per day is not specified. This prevents us from attributing a zero-pack-year history to a current smoker.

*Line 18* sets the value of ejection fraction (EF) to missing if it is entered as zero. Our database convention is to enter missing EF as zero in the database and to convert it to missing in the analysis program. An EF of zero is incompatible with life and would never be a true value.

*Lines 19–21* assign values to the indicator variables for EF quantiles as specified in the New York model.

*Line 22* assigns the value of 1 to the "EF missing" variable if EF is missing, and zero otherwise.

*Line 23* assigns the appropriate value to the variable for recent myocardial infarction (myocardial infarction that occurs in less than one week prior to surgery).

*Line 24* converts data we capture in the database, number of previous open-heart operations, to the New York model's requirement for previous operation 1 or 0.

*Line 25* sets the value of M70, the variable for the number of years above 70 years of age.

*Line 26* sets the value of M70 to zero if the patient's age is 70 or less to keep negative numbers from being assigned to M70.

*Line 27* sets the value of the variable "disaster" to 1 if the patient had an acute structural defect, renal failure or shock prior to surgery. Zero otherwise.

*Lines 28–32* calculate the odds of mortality from the New York State equation. The equation is taken from Table 4.2, which is reproduced with permission from *JAMA*.

*Line 33* converts mortality odds to probability.

*Line 34* raises probability from line 33 to percent.

*Line 35* submits all the statements above it.

*Lines 36 and 37* request the print that is shown as Table 4.5.

*Line 38* submits the print request.

# Appendix 2 Explanation of the program shown in Table 4.6

```
1  data oe;
2  input o e;
3  oeratio=o/e;
4  lci=(o*((1-(1/(9*o))-((1.96/3)*(sqrt(1/o))))**3))/e;
5  uci=((o+1)*((1-(1/(9*(o+1)))+((1.96/3)*(sqrt(1/(o+1)))))**3))/e;
6  x2=((o-e)**2)/e;
7  p=1-probchi(x2,1);
8  cards;
9  2 2.37
10 ;
11 run;
12 proc print;run;
```

*Line 1* names the data set.

*Line 2* inputs the variables *o* (observed) and *e* (expected);

*Line 3* computes the observed/expected ratio (*O/E* ratio).

*Line 4* computes the lower 95% confidence interval.

*Line 5* computes the upper 95% confidence interval.

*Line 6* computes the chi-square quantile.

*Line 7* computes the probability of the chi-square test.

*Line 8* tells SAS that the input data will start on the next line (since we are not reading in a big external file in this case).

*Line 9* shows the data, observed = 2 and expected = 2.37.

*Line 10* tells SAS that there are no more data to read in.

*Line 11* submits the statements.

*Line 12* requests the print shown in Table 4.7 and submits the request.

# Appendix 3 Line-by-line explanation of the program in Table 6.13

```
*imported from d:\safi\thorisk2.dbf;
data risk;set thorisk2;
format dos yymmdd2.;
format age 2.;
format ppe 3.1;
if dos ge 11323 and dos le 11687 then year=91;
if dos ge 11688 and dos le 12053 then year=92;
if dos ge 12054 and dos le 12418 then year=93;
if dos ge 12419 and dos le 12783 then year=94;
if dos ge 12784 and dos le 13148 then year=95;
if dos ge 13149 and dos le 13514 then year=96;
if dos ge 13515 and dos le 13879 then year=97;
if dos ge 13880 and dos le 14244 then year=98;
if age gt 0 and age le 59 then ageq=1;
if age ge 60 and age le 67 then ageq=2;
if age ge 68 and age le 72 then ageq=3;
if age ge 73 then ageq=4;
if edeath=1 then edeath2=1;else edeath2=2;
if ppe=1 then ppe2=1;else ppe2=2;
if ppl=1 then ppl2=1;else ppl2=2;
if taaaii=1 then taaaii2=1;
if taaaii=0 then taaaii2=2;
if taaaiii=1 then taaaiii2=1;
if taaaiii=0 then taaaiii2=2;
if copd=1 then copd2=1;
if copd=0 then copd2=2;
if acuted=1 then acute2=1;
if acuted=0 then acute2=2;
if diabetes=1 then diab2=1;
if diabetes=0 then diab2=2;
if htn=1 then htn2=1;
if htn=0 then htn2=2;
if prevabd=1 then prevabd2=1;
if prevabd=0 then prevabd2=2;
if rup=1 then rup2=1;
if rup=0 then rup2=2;
if renins=1 then renins2=1;
if renins=0 then renins2=2;
if prevtaaa=1 then prevtaa2=1;
if prevtaaa=0 then prevtaa2=2;
if atype='DESC' then desc=1;else desc=0;
if sex='F' or sex='f' then female=1;else female=0;
if female=1 then fem2=1;
if female=0 then fem2=2;
if preneuro ne 1;
run;
proc sort;by dos;run;
data risk2;
```

```
49 do dos=11323 to 14244 by 1;
50 o=exp(6.0061+(dos*-0.0007));
51 p=o/(1+o);
52 output;
53 end;
54 run;
55 proc sort;by dos;run;
56 data both;merge risk risk2;by dos;run;
57 goptions device=winprtg htext=1 ftext=swiss;
58 axis1 length=15 cm label=(a=90 r=0);
59 axis2 length=15 cm order=(11323 to 14244 by 365);
60 symbol v=dot i=rl;
61 proc gplot data=risk;plot age*dos / vaxis=axis1 haxis=axis2;
62 label age='Age';
63 label dos='Year of Operation';
64 run;
65 goptions device=winprtg htext=1 ftext=swiss;
66 axis1 length=15 cm label=(a=90 r=0) order=(0 to 1 by 0.1);
67 axis2 length=15 cm order=(11323 to 14244 by 365);
68 symbol v=dot i=none;
69 proc gplot data=risk;plot ppe*dos / vaxis=axis1 haxis=axis2;
70 label ppe='Occurrence of Neurologic Deficit';
71 label dos='Year of Operation';
72 run;
73 goptions device=winprtc htext=1 ftext=swiss;
74 axis1 length=15 cm label=(a=90 r=0) order=(0 to 1 by 0.1);
75 axis2 length=15 cm order=(11323 to 14244 by 365);
76 symbol2 v=dot i=none c=black;
77 symbol1 v=none i=join w=10 c=black;
78 proc gplot data=both;plot (p ppe)*dos / overlay vaxis=axis1 haxis=axis2;
79 label p='Probability of Neurologic Deficit';
80 label dos='Year of Operation';
81 run;
82 proc print;run;
83 run;
```

*Line 1* is a note that tells the programmer where the source data are located. Lines that begin with * are comment lines and they are ignored by SAS.

*Line 2* names the dataset, and subsets it from another dataset that has been imported from a dbase file. At the time we started this particular project there was no translation utility from Microsoft Access to SAS, so we had to export data to dbase files and import them into SAS that way. An advantage to reading data in from database files directly rather than from flat files is that the database will tell SAS the format and name of each variable, which does away with the input step. A disadvantage is that if the database file was not set up carefully variable formatting can be sub-optimal, and format statements may be required to get things into a form that can be reported easily.

*Lines 3–5* re-format date, age and neurological deficit (paraplegia or paraparesis) variables.

*Lines 6–13* convert SAS date values to year of surgery, which makes them easier to handle and interpret.
*Lines 14–17* divide age into quartiles.
*Lines 18–40* re-code variables from the standard 1 = yes 0 = no format to the 1 = yes 2 = no format that SAS requires for contingency table analysis.
*Line 41* creates a variable for descending thoracic aneurysm.
*Line 42* converts the character variable for gender to a 0–1 indicator variable for female gender.
*Lines 43 and 44* re-code female gender to 1,2 coding.
*Line 45* excludes any patients who had pre-existing paraplegia or paraparesis prior to surgery. We are interested only in incident cases, not prevalent ones.
*Line 46* submits the statements.
*Line 47* sorts the data by date of surgery.
*Line 48* creates a new dataset called risk 2.
*Line 49* creates date values for that dataset ranging over the exact period the actual study data cover. This is done to produce a scale variable for the slope that we will see in the next line.
*Line 50* calculates the odds of a neurological deficit across the entire range of dates of surgery using a logistic regression equation for probability of neurological deficit over time.
*Line 51* computes the probability (risk) from the odds.
*Line 52* outputs the iterated data.
*Line 53* ends the do loop.
*Line 54* submits the statements.
*Line 55* sorts the outputted probability calculations by date.
*Line 56* merges the calculated data with the actual data from the previous dataset by date of surgery.
*Line 57* sets the general graphics options for the first plot (which appears as Figure 6.2). It specifies that the device is a Windows grayscale printer (a black and white laser printer), that the height of the text = 1 and the font of the text is swiss.
*Lines 58 and 59* set the axis parameters for the first plot, including their length, the orientation of the labels, and their range and order.
*Line 60* defines the plot characters (a dot for the value of each observation and a linear regression line).
*Line 61* requests a plot of age by date of surgery and identifies the axis commands from lines 58 and 59.
*Lines 62 and 63* show the text for the labels.
*Line 64* submits the statement.
*Lines 65–72* request essentially the same things as lines 57–64, but for the plot of neurological deficit occurrence versus date of surgery. This plot appears as Figure 6.3.
*Lines 73–81* do the same for the next plot (Figure 6.4). The main difference here is in *line*

*78*, where the plot statement reads in data from the iterative dataset we created using the logistic regression equation in lines 48–54. Here, the plot statement requests a plot of (p ppe)*dos, where p = probability from the logistic equation, ppe = presence or absence of neurological deficit, and dos = date of surgery. We iterated the probability estimate across the exact date of surgery range so we could match the calculated probability with the actual data of occurrence of the deficits. When two dependent variables are to be plotted against one independent variable on one plot, the overlay option is specified so the plots will be combined.

*Line 82* requests a print and runs it.

# Index